Meditative Heartbeat Therapy

A CONTEMPLATIVE GUIDE TO PRESENCE, RHYTHM, AND CARE AT THE END OF LIFE

DANIEL DELOMA

APOCRYPHILE
PRESS

Apocryphile Press
PO Box 255
Hannacroix, NY 12087
www.apocryphilepress.com

The author would like to thank Janeen Jones for her excellent editing.

Please join our mailing list at www.apocryphilepress.com/free. We'll keep you up-to-date on all our new releases, and we'll also send you a FREE BOOK. Visit us today!

CONTENTS

Acknowledgments   vii

A Note to the Reader   ix

PART ONE
ORIGINS AND BACKGROUND

1. Welcome to Meditative Heartbeat Therapy (MHbT)   3
2. The Role of MHbT in Palliative and End-of-Life Care   8

   Reflection   12
   The Heartbeat as a Bridge Between Life and Death

3. Theoretical and Practical Foundations of MHbT   17

   Reflection   28
   Embodying the Rhythm of Life

PART TWO
SPIRITUAL, ETHICAL, AND PHILOSOPHICAL FOUNDATIONS

4. The Spiritual Foundations of Meditative Heartbeat Therapy   35

   Reflection   41
   One Rhythm, One Life—A Meditation on the Sacred Heartbeat

5. The Breath of the Soul   45

   Reflection   59
   The Body's Last Offering

6. The Heart and the Bardo   60

   Reflection   64
   Thresholds, Echoes, and the Unfinished Song

7. Ethical Considerations and Challenges in Implementing MHbT   66

   Reflection   71

8. Cultural Diversity in Spiritual Integration and MHbT   76

   Reflection   117
   The Power of Stories in Healing and Transformation

PART THREE
CLINICAL APPLICATIONS

9. Integrative Palliative Care and MHbT   125
   Reflection   136
   The Rhythm That Binds Us
10. Integrating MHbT, Reiki, and Clinical Hypnosis   139
    Reflection   145
    The Rhythm of Healing
11. Palliative Clinical Hypnosis and MHbT   149
    Reflection   157
    The Doorway Between Worlds
12. Incorporating MHbT into End-of-Life Doula Practice   160
    Reflection   169
    The Sacred Rhythm of Life and Death
13. Breath and Flame: Integrating MHbT with
    Supplemental Oxygen   171
    Reflection   190
    This Merciful Machine
14. Other Practical Applications of MHbT   199
    Reflection   203
    The Rhythm That Connects Us All

Conclusion   207
and Reflections on the Journey of MHbT

Bibliography   213
Appendix   215

For the hundreds of heartbeats I was privileged to hear —
the ones whose rhythm gave these words life.
Though they have faded from the physical world,
they now ride on the breath of the trees,
and their voices are woven into these pages.

ACKNOWLEDGMENTS

This work is woven from the rhythms of many hearts, and I offer my deepest thanks to those who have walked beside me in its unfolding.

To *Kathy Maraia, Sylvia Brockman*, and *Mary Ross* — your wisdom, encouragement, and presence shaped this work in ways both subtle and profound. I carry your guidance with me in every beat.

To *Rev. Dr. Paula Belleggie* — your teachings on sacred accompaniment and embodied theology continue to echo through my practice and my pages.

To *John Mabry* — thank you for believing in the heart of this work and for welcoming it into the Apocryphile family with such care and spirit. Your own path of deep inquiry inspires me.

To *Janeen Jones* — thank you for the gift of your attentive eye and steady hand. Your care has helped this work find its truest voice.

To the teams at *Waveny LifeCare Network, The Integrative Palliative Care Institute*, and *Fairfield University*, thank you for the ways you continue to hold space for innovation, healing, and contemplative presence in palliative care.

To *St. Christopher's Hospice*, whose global fellowship and contemplative care teachings deepened this work — I am grateful for the insight and community you have offered from the very birthplace of modern hospice.

To the *Pequot Museum and Research Center*, and the *Pequot Library of Southport, Connecticut* — your preservation of sacred rhythm, memory, and spirit helped ground this work in history and living tradition.

And to the countless patients, caregivers, and colleagues who shared their breath, their stories, and their heartbeats — this work is for you. Your presence lives on in every pulse, every silence, and every sacred rhythm that follows.

A NOTE TO THE READER

In the quiet hours of sitting beside the dying, I have often wondered: what truly comforts us at the edge of life? What do we reach for—not just physically, but spiritually—when language fades, when pain lingers, when time stretches thin?

Meditative Heartbeat Therapy (MHbT) arose from that wondering. It emerged not from theory, but from presence—built through years of interdisciplinary hospice work, spiritual care, and contemplative listening. It is a response to a growing need: for integrative, soul-centered approaches that attend to the whole person—mind, body, and spirit—without abandoning the clinical grounding that ensures safety and efficacy.

This work is not a rejection of medicine, but a rebalancing. It invites us to remember that we are rhythmic creatures—beating, breathing, bound by pulse and breath to the living world around us. MHbT is a therapy, yes—but it is also a theology, a philosophy, and a way of being with the dying that affirms the sacredness of the body even as the spirit prepares to let go.

The intention of this book is not to suggest that pain is anything other than physical. Rather, it is to acknowledge that reality while affirming the truth that, as embodied and spiritual beings, physical pain inevitably gives rise to spiritual distress. Meditative Heartbeat Therapy is offered as a way of easing that distress—even amid profound physical suffering—while complementing medical and pharmacological interventions.

The chapters that follow move between the practical and the poetic, the clinical and the contemplative. They include evidence-based applications, case studies, and ritual elements—woven together to offer both guidance and grounding. Whether you are a clinician, a caregiver, a chaplain, or a seeker, may you find in these pages a rhythm that resonates with your own.

Finally, dear reader, I urge you to go forth not merely listening to the words of those in your care, but to the quiet, persistent rhythm of their hearts. Especially during the most sacred threshold—the final 72 hours—listen with reverence. Let each heartbeat echo not just in time, but through eternity.

—Daniel DeLoma

PART ONE
ORIGINS AND BACKGROUND

Every therapy has a beginning, but Meditative Heartbeat Therapy began not in a lab or classroom, but at the bedside—where breath slows, where silence thickens, where the human presence itself becomes the medicine. In this opening section, we trace the emergence of MHbT through lived experience, spiritual discernment, and clinical necessity. These chapters lay the philosophical and theological groundwork for the work that follows. Here, we explore the sacred importance of rhythm, of the body as a vessel, and of presence as the first and most lasting form of care. The reader is invited not only to understand the birth of MHbT, but to begin to feel its pulse.

WELCOME TO MEDITATIVE HEARTBEAT THERAPY (MHBT)

There is a rhythm beneath everything. Before the first cry, before the first word, even before the breath—there is the heartbeat. It is the earliest music of our existence. And when the breath returns to silence, the heartbeat becomes the last sound echoing through the body. Between those two sacred thresholds, we live. And there, within that span, Meditative Heartbeat Therapy finds its voice.

In countless rooms, I sat at the bedside of the dying. I felt the stillness of a moment held between heartbeats. I have heard the breath catch, resume, soften. I have seen a single hand resting lightly over a chest, the faint tap of pulse beneath palm, offering reassurance when words fail. These are the spaces where Meditative Heartbeat Therapy (MHbT) was born—not in a lab or a lecture hall, but in the quiet presence between people.

MHbT is a spiritually rooted, clinically grounded integrative approach to end-of-life care that uses the natural rhythm of the heartbeat as an anchor for presence, comfort, and spiritual exploration. It pairs recorded heartbeat sounds with guided breathing, sacred silence, or intentional bedside ritual. It is not a replacement for medicine, but a companion to it. An integrative care in the truest sense. It meets the patient not with intervention, not with invasiveness, but with reverence.

In a world where care at the end of life is often fragmented, overly clinical, or spiritually impoverished, MHbT seeks to restore wholeness. It invites clinicians, caregivers, chaplains, doulas, family members, and patients themselves to return to the most primal language that we share: rhythm. It reminds us that we do not need to invent healing—we only need to remember how to listen.

Consider this the first embrace—a gentle unfolding of the philosophy and framework behind the practice. But it is also a declaration: that dying is not a medical failure. It is a spiritual threshold. And it deserves more than sedation and silence—it deserves presence.

THE ORIGIN STORY: WHERE RHYTHM BEGAN

It began with a patient—a man in his early 80s, curled quietly beneath a thin blanket, eyes closed, breath shallow. He had been unresponsive for several hours. His daughter sat nearby, softly crying, unsure if he could hear her. She held his hand, stroked his hair, whispered memories. Nothing changed.

I asked gently, "Would it be alright if I offered a moment of shared breath?" She nodded. I placed my stethoscope against his chest and let her listen. "That's your dad's heartbeat," I said. "That's the rhythm he's carried his whole life." Her tears changed. They softened. She smiled.

I recorded the sound as best I could with the rudimentary technology that I had on hand and let it play softly from the poor quality speakers on my phone as we sat in silence. Despite the technology not being perfect, the atmosphere shifted. The room didn't feel medical anymore. It felt holy. He didn't wake. He didn't need to. The rhythm had returned him to his body—and returned her to him.

That moment became the seed of a practice. I began to explore ways to bring heartbeat-based meditation into hospice and palliative care. I partnered with nurses, social workers, chaplains, music therapists, and doulas. And over time, a simple act of listening became something larger.

As more people welcomed the practice into the room, it took on a life of its own. Nurses noticed patients with terminal restlessness settling more quickly. Chaplains found that patients who resisted traditional prayer could open to the wordless comfort of rhythm. Family members, unsure of what to say in their loved ones' final hours, began to sit and simply breathe together—matching the beat, holding vigil in sound and silence.

WHAT IS MEDITATIVE HEARTBEAT THERAPY?

MHbT is both profoundly simple and infinitely adaptable.

At its core, the practice involves using the sound (or sensation) of a steady heartbeat—recorded, remembered, or imagined—as a focal point for meditation, comfort, and spiritual grounding. That sound is paired with intentional presence, guided breathing, silence, prayer, and/or ritual, depending on the setting and needs of the patient.

Clinically, MHbT can:

- Reduce anxiety and agitation
- Help regulate breath and pulse through entrainment
- Offer spiritual grounding during times of physical and emotional distress
- Provide a nonverbal anchor for patients with dementia or language barriers

Spiritually, it can:

- Create a sacred container for dying
- Reconnect patients to the rhythm of life
- Serve as a ritual of return—for patient and family alike
- Invite the soul to feel seen, held, and heard

MHbT is used in a variety of settings:

- *In hospice units*, as part of integrative comfort care
- *In private homes*, guided by doulas, clinicians, or spiritual companions
- *In hospitals*, adapted for palliative chaplaincy or bereavement care
- *In caregiver support programs*, as a mindfulness and grounding tool

It requires no expensive equipment, no invasive procedures, and no dogma. Only presence, rhythm, and a willingness to listen.

MHbT also extends beyond the bedside. It can be used in grief groups, caregiver circles, and rituals of remembrance. It offers an avenue for families to reconnect with the memory of their loved one's presence—not just through photos or recordings, but through rhythm, which lives on long after sound has ceased.

WHY THE HEARTBEAT?

Because it is the first sound.
Because it is the last sound.
Because it is the one thing no one needs to be taught how to feel.

The heartbeat bypasses language and cognition. It calls to something older. Something cellular. In nearly every culture and tradition, rhythm has been used to enter sacred space. From drumming circles to monastic chants to the slow chant of "Om," rhythm has always been a bridge between worlds. MHbT is that same bridge, offered at the end of life.

There's also neuroscience to consider: rhythmic auditory stimuli can entrain neural patterns, regulate the autonomic nervous system, and offer comfort in chaos. But MHbT is not just about neurobiology. It's about allowing people to *feel* like themselves again—like they are still someone, even in their dying.

It is true that this book is written for clinicians, caregivers, chaplains, end-of-life doulas, nurses, and anyone who walks with the dying. But it is also written for those who grieve. For those who remember a heartbeat they can no longer hear. For those who feel the absence of the body as deeply as the presence of the soul. It is written for anyone who has ever asked, "How do I help?" and been told there's nothing to be done.

Because there is always something to be done.

You can listen. You can breathe. You can hold rhythm. You can sit in silence and let the soul remember the sound of itself.

That is more than enough. That is holy.

In the chapters ahead, you will find:

- The clinical foundations and theoretical frameworks that support MHbT
- The spiritual and cultural roots that give it shape
- Real-world applications, case studies, and patient stories
- Reflections that invite you to internalize what you're learning
- Tools to begin offering MHbT in your setting or home

You do not need to be a healer, a minister, or a mystic. You only need to be human. And to believe that presence matters.

MHbT is not a method reserved for specialists. It is a return to the most ancient form of care: *to sit, to breathe, to listen.*

Welcome to Meditative Heartbeat Therapy.
Let us listen together.

CHAPTER 2

THE ROLE OF MHBT IN PALLIATIVE AND END-OF-LIFE CARE

MHbT is a therapeutic technique that taps into the meditative power of a natural bodily rhythm: the heartbeat. The therapy reflects a broader trend in palliative care that emphasizes spiritual and emotional well-being, addressing existential fears in patients who are nearing the end of life. By anchoring attention on the heartbeat, MHbT allows patients to cultivate presence, reducing anxiety and promoting acceptance.

Holistic interventions are increasingly essential in palliative care because they address nonphysical suffering, such as fear of death and emotional isolation. The heartbeat serves as a bridge between the physical and spiritual, grounding the patient in their bodily experience while opening pathways to deeper reflection on life's meaning. This process fosters peace, helping individuals confront the unknown with grace.

The integration of mindfulness into healthcare can be traced back to the 1970s. Over the past few decades, these practices have transitioned from stress-reduction clinics into mainstream healthcare settings, including oncology, mental health services, and hospice care. Mindfulness practices have become essential tools for managing chronic conditions and supporting patients in end-of-life transitions.

In hospice care, the emphasis has shifted from curative treatments to comfort-focused care. Mindfulness aligns with this focus, as it encourages patients to remain present, fostering acceptance of life as it unfolds. Early studies highlighted the potential for mindfulness to reduce pain perception, manage anxiety, and enhance emotional stability.

MHbT builds upon these foundational principles but takes a more personalized approach by focusing on the rhythm of the heartbeat. This personal rhythm becomes a unique meditative anchor, offering both symbolic and sensory comfort. According to research, mindfulness practices tailored to specific experiences—like listening to one's heartbeat—are particularly effective in palliative care.

THE NEED FOR NON-PHARMACOLOGICAL INTERVENTIONS IN HOSPICE

The reliance on medications for symptom management in palliative care can create challenges, including side effects that diminish the patient's quality of life. Non-pharmacological interventions such as MHbT offer integrative benefits, addressing psychological and emotional suffering without the risks associated with medication. Benzodiazepines, commonly prescribed to manage anxiety, can cause cognitive impairment, drowsiness, and dependency, underscoring the need for alternatives.

Studies in palliative settings suggest that spiritual and emotional distress contribute significantly to patients' suffering. For example, existential anxiety—the fear of death, meaninglessness, and isolation—is common among hospice patients. MHbT provides a pathway for patients to explore these fears, fostering emotional reconciliation and acceptance through focused meditation.

Integrating MHbT into care plans also reduces caregiver burden, as patients who engage in non-pharmacological therapies often require fewer interventions for emotional crises. This dual benefit ensures better resource management while enhancing patient well-being. Systematic reviews of mindfulness interventions have shown a reduction in caregiver burden and an increase in emotional resilience among both patients and healthcare workers.

EMOTIONAL AND SPIRITUAL COMFORT THROUGH MHBT

The heartbeat serves as a powerful metaphor for life's continuity. In MHbT sessions, patients are encouraged to focus on this rhythm, creating a sense of presence that transcends immediate distress. This practice aligns with theories of existential psychology, which suggest that confronting mortality with presence can transform fear into peace.

Many patients describe MHbT as a spiritual experience, interpreting the heartbeat as a sign of connection to a larger life force or divine presence. This reflective state allows them to revisit significant life experiences and cultivate gratitude for meaningful moments. The act of listening deeply to the heartbeat fosters a meditative state where unresolved emotions can surface and be processed.

In a hospice context, where patients often grapple with issues of legacy and meaning, MHbT offers an opportunity for deep personal reflection. For instance, patients may reflect on relationships, unfinished goals, or personal achievements during sessions. Practitioners play a crucial role in facilitating these reflections, ensuring that patients feel safe and supported throughout the process. The positive feedback loop created by these reflective sessions promotes emotional well-being, even as physical health declines.

MHbT offers a new paradigm for end-of-life care, emphasizing the importance of spiritual and emotional well-being alongside physical comfort. By focusing on the heartbeat, this therapy creates a bridge between the tangible and intangible aspects of human experience, helping patients navigate the complexities of their final days with grace.

The integration of MHbT into palliative care plans demonstrates the potential for non-pharmacological therapies to enhance quality of life. As healthcare systems continue to embrace holistic care models, interventions like MHbT will play an increasingly vital role in supporting patients and caregivers alike. Through interdisciplinary collaboration and personalized care, MHbT ensures that patients can experience their final journey with dignity, peace, and acceptance.

REFLECTION

THE HEARTBEAT AS A BRIDGE
BETWEEN LIFE AND DEATH

In the quiet moments of our lives, how often do we pause to listen—to truly listen—to the steady rhythm of our own heartbeat? It is a sound so familiar that we rarely acknowledge it, a presence so constant that it recedes into the background of our awareness. And yet, it is the first sound we hear in the womb and the last rhythm to leave us in death. It is our earliest tether to life, our most enduring companion, and our final surrender.

Change is not to be feared but embraced—that impermanence is not a failing of existence but its essence. Our heartbeat, like the tides and the turning of the seasons, reminds us of this truth. It rises and falls, quickens and slows, mirroring the fluid nature of our lives. To listen to our heartbeat is to accept that all things—our joys, our sorrows, our very selves—exist only for a time. Yet within that fleeting existence, there is a profound beauty, an invitation to be present to the gift of now.

In end-of-life care, this understanding takes on an even deeper significance. For those standing at the threshold between life and death, the heartbeat is a final, steady presence, a reminder that even in the face of uncertainty, life continues—beat by beat, breath by breath. Meditative Heartbeat Therapy (MHbT) offers not just comfort, but a way to be fully here in this moment, allowing both patients and their loved ones to meet life's final transition with dignity, with grace, and with peace.

To listen—truly listen—is a radical and sacred act. In a world filled with distractions and demands, we rarely offer our full attention to anything, least of all to the quiet rhythms of our own being. Yet MHbT places listening at the very heart of healing. It asks nothing of us except to be present, to attune ourselves to the sound of life itself and to welcome whatever arises.

For those facing the end of life, this act of listening creates space for deep reflection. No longer striving or resisting, they are invited to simply be—with their heartbeat, with their emotions, with the fullness of their experience. Grief, fear, love, and longing may all surface, but rather than being overwhelming, these emotions are held within the steady rhythm of the heart. In this way, MHbT offers a path toward reconciliation—not through words, but through presence.

What have we carried with us through this life? What stories have shaped us? What remains unresolved? As the sound of the heartbeat becomes a mirror, these questions emerge, not as burdens, but as invitations—to forgive, to release, to celebrate, and to honor the journey we have walked.

For caregivers, this practice is equally transformative. To listen to a patient's heartbeat alongside them is to enter into a profound communion—one that does not require speech, only presence. It is a reminder that, at our core, we are all moving through this life together, bound by the same rhythms of existence.

In times of transition—birth, love, loss, and death—we often find ourselves searching for meaning. What lies beyond the limits of what we know? Where do we go when we leave this world?

For some, the heartbeat is more than a biological rhythm; it is a spiritual presence, a link to something greater than themselves. Some patients describe hearing their heartbeat as a connection to the love of those who have gone before them. Others feel it as a pulse of the divine, a reminder that they are not separate but part of something vast and enduring.

We should not demand certainty in matters of the soul, but rather invite each person to seek their own understanding of life's great mysteries. In MHbT, patients are given the space to explore these questions on their own terms. Whether they find comfort in faith, in love, or simply in the beauty of existence itself, the heartbeat remains a steady companion, guiding them toward whatever lies beyond.

For those left behind, the absence of a heartbeat is a silence that can feel unbearable. The loss of that familiar rhythm—a rhythm we once held close, felt in an embrace, heard in the quiet of the night—can be a painful reminder of what is gone. And yet, if we listen closely, we may find that their rhythm has not vanished.

It is in the wind that moves through the trees, in the ocean's gentle waves, in the quiet breathing of those who remain. The rhythm of a life does not simply disappear; it lingers in the memories we hold, the love we share, and the ways in which we continue to honor those who have shaped our journey.

Many families who experience MHbT as part of the dying process find solace in this continuity. Some choose to record the heartbeat of their loved one, preserving it as a sacred reminder of their presence. Others weave the memory of that sound into their grief rituals—listening to it during times of remembrance, integrating it into meditation, or simply recalling it in moments of longing. In this way, the heartbeat becomes more than a sound; it becomes a bridge between past and present, a symbol of the love that endures beyond physical separation.

At the heart of all spiritual traditions is the lesson of surrender—not as a passive resignation, but as an active and courageous trust in the unfolding of life. MHbT teaches this lesson in its simplest and most profound form. When we listen to the heartbeat, we do not control its rhythm; we follow it. We do not dictate its pace; we surrender to its natural flow.

For those at the end of life, this practice becomes a way of preparing for the final letting go. In tuning into the heartbeat, they begin to understand that life itself has always been a process of release. We release childhood to enter adulthood. We release one breath to take in the next. We release the day to welcome the night. Death, then, is not an interruption of life's rhythm—it is its final, inevitable movement.

To let go is not to be defeated, but to trust. It is to understand that we are held in something greater than ourselves—a vast and inter-woven web of existence that does not end, but only changes form. Unitarian Universalism teaches us that while we may not know what comes after death, we can trust in the love and meaning that we have cultivated in life. MHbT offers a way to embody that trust, to practice surrendering moment by moment, until the final release becomes not a fearful leap, but a natural step in the dance of existence.

For caregivers, too, there is a lesson in this surrender. They learn that their role is not to fix, not to prevent, but to accompany. To be a witness. To offer presence. There is an immense grace in under-standing that being there—truly, wholly there—is enough.

And in the end, what remains of a life? Is it the words we spoke? The things we accomplished? Or is it something deeper, something more elemental?

Perhaps our greatest legacy is not in what we did, but in how we were present. The way we showed up for others. The way we listened, loved, and shared our lives. The way our heartbeat, however briefly, touched the lives of those around us.

The practice of MHbT teaches us that presence is a gift—not just at the end of life, but in all the moments leading up to it. If we can learn to listen to the heartbeat now, to be present with ourselves and with one another in the midst of daily life, then we are already preparing for a good death. A death where nothing is left unsaid, where love has been fully given, where we can surrender in peace.

And so, as we step forward from this reflection, let us take with us the lessons of the heartbeat. Let us listen more deeply—to ourselves, to each other, to the life that moves through us all. Let us embrace the fleeting nature of existence, not with fear, but with gratitude. Let us surrender to the rhythm of life, trusting that it will carry us where we need to go.

And when the time comes, as it will for each of us, may we meet that final beat not with resistance, but with reverence. Knowing that even as one rhythm fades, the great song of life continues.

CHAPTER 3

THEORETICAL
AND PRACTICAL
FOUNDATIONS OF MHBT

A s stated in Chapter 1, The genesis of Meditative Heartbeat Therapy did not emerge from a laboratory or a policy meeting. It arose, instead, from the profoundly intimate act of sitting at the bedside of a dying person. The original insights were quiet, observed rather than declared—rooted in sound, silence, and story. This chapter further traces that origin. Before we speak of methodology, we must speak of meaning. Before we systematize, we must listen.

UNDERSTANDING THE ROLE OF
HEARTBEAT AWARENESS IN EMOTIONAL REGULATION

Meditative Heartbeat Therapy (MHbT) utilizes the heartbeat as a grounding anchor for emotional regulation. This concept is rooted in the understanding that the heartbeat is one of the most fundamental and continuous experiences of the body. It is a constant reminder of life and existence, creating a direct line to the present moment.

When individuals face emotional distress—be it anxiety, fear, grief, or sadness—focusing on the heartbeat can help them stabilize their emotional states. The process involves:

1. *Physiological Anchoring*: The heartbeat serves as a physiological anchor that helps individuals transition from a state of heightened emotional arousal to one of calmness and relaxation. Studies have shown that when individuals engage in heartbeat awareness, they often experience a decrease in physiological symptoms of anxiety, such as elevated heart rates and rapid breathing.

2. *Mindfulness and Presence*: By concentrating on their heartbeat, patients practice mindfulness, a technique that encourages individuals to be present in the moment without judgment. This practice has been linked to numerous psychological benefits, including reduced stress and improved emotional resilience.

3. *Emotional Processing*: Engaging with one's heartbeat provides a unique avenue for emotional processing. Patients can explore their feelings in a safe and structured manner, allowing for the acknowledgment and acceptance of complex emotions.

Consider the case of David, a 63-year-old man diagnosed with advanced lung cancer. Upon entering hospice care, David expressed feelings of deep anxiety and fear surrounding his diagnosis. His healthcare team introduced him to MHbT, beginning with simple heartbeat awareness exercises.

- *Initial Reactions*: Initially resistant to the idea, David found it difficult to focus on his heartbeat amidst his anxious thoughts. However, through guided sessions, he gradually learned to anchor himself to the rhythmic sound of his heart.

- *Gradual Transformation*: Over time, David reported feeling more in control of his anxiety. He stated, "Focusing on my heartbeat helps me remember that I'm still alive. It's comforting to have something constant to hold onto."

This transformation highlights the profound impact that heartbeat awareness can have on emotional regulation, illustrating the therapeutic potential of MHbT.

The connection between heartbeat awareness and emotional regulation can be elucidated through several psychological mechanisms:

- *Interoception*: Interoception is the body's ability to perceive internal signals, including heartbeat, hunger, and pain. By tuning into their heartbeat, patients enhance their interoceptive awareness, allowing them to recognize and understand their emotional responses better. This self-awareness is critical for emotional regulation, as it enables individuals to identify when they are becoming overwhelmed and to implement coping strategies proactively.
- *Mindfulness*: Mindfulness practices encourage individuals to observe their thoughts and feelings without judgment. When patients focus on their heartbeat, they engage in a form of mindfulness that helps them cultivate nonjudgmental awareness of their emotional states. This practice reduces reactivity to negative emotions and fosters a sense of acceptance.
- *Cognitive Reappraisal*: Listening to one's heartbeat can facilitate cognitive reappraisal, a strategy that involves reinterpreting a situation to alter its emotional impact. For example, a patient may initially feel fear at the thought of their heartbeat signaling impending death. However, through the lens of heartbeat awareness, they may come to see their heartbeat as a reminder of life and connection, shifting their emotional experience from fear to acceptance.

The practice of engaging with one's heartbeat not only aids emotional regulation but also contributes to overall psychological well-being. The following benefits have been documented in patients who regularly practice MHbT:

- *Reduced Anxiety*: Many patients report lower levels of anxiety after engaging in heartbeat awareness exercises. The rhythmic sound of their heart can serve as a soothing presence, helping them manage feelings of panic or fear.
- *Improved Emotional Resilience*: By regularly practicing MHbT, patients often develop greater emotional resilience. They learn to respond to distressing thoughts and feelings with compassion rather than judgment, leading to healthier coping mechanisms.
- *Enhanced Quality of Life*: Overall, individuals who engage with their heartbeat through MHbT report improvements in their quality of life. They express a greater sense of peace, acceptance, and connection with themselves and their loved ones.

Polyvagal Theory, developed by Dr. Stephen Porges, offers a compelling framework for understanding the impact of the autonomic nervous system on emotional regulation. According to this theory, the vagus nerve plays a crucial role in how individuals respond to stress and social interactions.

- *Ventral Vagal Complex (VVC)*: The VVC is associated with feelings of safety and social connection. When the VVC is activated, individuals are more likely to engage in social interactions and emotional connections. Listening to one's heartbeat through MHbT can stimulate the VVC, promoting feelings of safety and reducing anxiety.
- *Sympathetic Nervous System (SNS)*: The SNS is responsible for the "fight or flight" response, leading to increased heart rate and heightened emotional arousal. In situations of stress, the SNS becomes dominant, potentially leading to panic and distress. MHbT provides a counterbalance to

this response by grounding individuals in their heartbeat, helping them return to a state of calm.

The concept of embodied cognition posits that our thoughts, feelings, and behaviors are deeply intertwined with our physical experiences. This theory suggests that the body is not merely a vessel for the mind but an integral component of how individuals perceive and respond to their environments.

In MHbT, the focus on heartbeat awareness allows patients to reconnect with their bodies. This embodied approach facilitates emotional processing, as patients learn to recognize how their emotions manifest physically. For instance, a patient may notice that their heartbeat quickens when they feel anxious or that it slows when they feel at peace. This awareness can help them develop strategies to manage their emotional responses more effectively.

THE ROLE OF THE HEART IN EMOTIONAL AND SPIRITUAL HEALTH

The heart has long been considered a symbol of emotion and connection. In many cultures, it represents love, compassion, and the essence of being. Understanding the symbolic significance of the heart can enhance the practice of MHbT, allowing patients to explore their emotional and spiritual landscapes more profoundly.

CULTURAL PERSPECTIVES

- *Indigenous Wisdom*: Many Indigenous cultures view the heart as the center of emotional and spiritual life. Heartbeat meditation aligns with these perspectives, fostering a deep sense of connection to oneself and the universe.
- *Eastern Philosophies*: In many Eastern philosophies, the heart is seen as a source of wisdom and intuition. Practices

that focus on the heart, such as *Heartfulness Meditation*, resonate with the principles of MHbT, reinforcing the importance of heart-centered awareness.

MHbT offers a unique intersection between psychology and spirituality, addressing both emotional and spiritual dimensions of well-being. Patients often find themselves grappling with existential questions as they approach the end of life. Through heartbeat awareness, they can explore these questions in a safe and supportive environment.

Practitioners can encourage patients to reflect on the symbolic meaning of their heartbeat. Questions such as "What does your heartbeat remind you of?" or "How do you feel connected to your life journey through your heartbeat?" can prompt profound spiritual insights.

For instance, when working with a patient named Grace, who was nearing the end of her life, the practitioner encouraged her to engage in heartbeat meditation. As Grace listened to her heartbeat, she began to reflect on her life's journey, leading to feelings of gratitude and acceptance. "Listening to my heart reminds me of all the love I've experienced," she stated, illustrating the profound spiritual insights that can arise through MHbT.

The emotional benefits of MHbT are profound. Patients report that listening to their heartbeat provides a sense of comfort and grounding, particularly in the face of distressing emotions. MHbT can help with:

- *Emotional Validation*: Engaging with one's heartbeat allows patients to acknowledge and validate their emotions. Rather than suppressing feelings of fear or sadness, they learn to observe them without judgment.
- *Fostering Acceptance*: Through repeated practice, patients often develop a sense of acceptance regarding their emotional states. They come to understand that emotions

are a natural part of the human experience, leading to greater self-compassion.

Consider the journey of Sarah, a 55-year-old woman with terminal cancer. During her initial sessions, Sarah expressed feelings of overwhelming sadness and fear. As she engaged with MHbT, she discovered that listening to her heartbeat offered a sense of solace. "It's like my heart is reminding me that I'm still here, still alive," she reflected. Over time, Sarah learned to use heartbeat meditation as a tool for emotional regulation, helping her navigate her feelings with greater ease.

In addition to emotional benefits, MHbT provides a platform for spiritual exploration. Many patients find themselves grappling with existential questions and seeking meaning as they face the end of life. Listening to their heartbeat can evoke feelings of connection to something greater than themselves.

Practitioners often encourage patients to reflect on the symbolic meaning of their heartbeat. Questions such as "What does your heartbeat tell you about your journey?" or "How does this rhythm connect you to your loved ones?" can prompt profound spiritual insights.

One poignant example involves Robert, a 72-year-old man facing advanced prostate cancer. During his MHbT sessions, Robert began to reflect on the memories associated with his heartbeat—the births of his children, the laughter shared with friends, and the quiet moments spent in nature. He expressed, "Each beat feels like a reminder of all the love I've known." This exploration allowed Robert to cultivate a sense of peace as he approached the end of his life.

Family members also play a crucial role in the MHbT process. Joint sessions where family members listen to a loved one's heartbeat create opportunities for emotional intimacy and shared healing. This familial support enhances the overall therapeutic experience, allowing families to engage in meaningful conversations about life, love, and loss.

Practitioners can facilitate family-centered MHbT sessions by creating a safe space for open communication. This involves establishing ground rules for sharing, encouraging vulnerability, and fostering empathy among family members.

CASE EXAMPLE: HEALING TOGETHER

In a family session, the Johnson family gathered around their matriarch, Grace, who was nearing the end of her life. As they listened to her heartbeat together, they began to share stories of their favorite memories with her. This experience fostered emotional closeness, allowing them to express gratitude and love. Grace remarked, "Hearing all of your voices while listening to my heartbeat makes me feel so alive." This shared experience highlighted the power of MHbT to create connections among family members.

PRACTICAL APPLICATIONS OF MHBT

Individual MHbT Sessions. The structure of individual MHbT sessions is vital for fostering a safe space for patients. Practitioners can adapt their approach based on the patient's needs, ensuring that each session is tailored to support their emotional and spiritual journeys. Here is a sample session structure:

1. *Introduction*: Begin with a warm greeting and a brief discussion about the patient's emotional state.
2. *Grounding Exercise*: Engage in breath awareness or a calming visualization to help the patient relax.
3. *Heartbeat Listening*: Record the patient's heartbeat and play it back, encouraging them to focus on the sound.
4. *Reflective Discussion*: Use open-ended questions to facilitate exploration of emotions and experiences.
5. *Closing Reflection*: Summarize the session and encourage the patient to journal about their experience.

Family-Centered MHbT Sessions. Family-centered sessions can help enhance emotional bonds among family members while allowing them to support the patient in their journey. Practitioners should create an inclusive environment that encourages open communication and connection. Here is a sample family session structure:

1. *Introduction*: Welcome family members and discuss the goals of the session.
2. *Joint Grounding Exercise*: Facilitate synchronized breathing or mindfulness techniques as a family.
3. *Heartbeat Listening*: Play the recording of the patient's heartbeat, encouraging shared focus and reflection.
4. *Family Reflection*: Invite family members to share their thoughts and feelings about the experience.
5. *Closing Ritual*: Conclude with a shared affirmation or moment of silence, reinforcing family unity.

INDIVIDUAL CASE STUDY: HEALING THROUGH HEARTBEAT AWARENESS

John, a 70-year-old man diagnosed with metastatic prostate cancer, faced significant emotional challenges as he transitioned into hospice care. He struggled with feelings of hopelessness and despair, finding it difficult to connect with his family and express his emotions.

The hospice team introduced MHbT as part of John's care plan. During the first session, the practitioner guided him through a heartbeat meditation. John listened to a recording of his heartbeat and reflected on the emotions that arose.

Over the course of several sessions, John reported feeling increasingly connected to himself and his loved ones. He began to articulate his feelings and share stories with his family during their visits. "Listening to my heartbeat reminds me that I'm still here, still part of this family," he shared, illustrating the emotional healing that MHbT facilitated.

FAMILY CASE STUDY:
RECONNECTING WITH HEARTBEAT THERAPY

The Garcia family faced the impending loss of their patriarch, Miguel, who had been diagnosed with advanced liver cancer. The family struggled with grief, fear, and unresolved conflicts that had surfaced over the years.

The hospice team organized family-centered MHbT sessions, encouraging the Garcias to engage in heartbeat meditation together. They listened to Miguel's heartbeat and shared reflections about their relationships.

Through these shared experiences, the family members began to reconnect emotionally. They expressed feelings of love and appreciation, leading to moments of forgiveness and understanding. Miguel stated, "Listening to my heartbeat together helps us remember what truly matters—our love for each other."

Advancements in technology offer exciting possibilities for enhancing the practice of MHbT. Potential avenues include:

- *Mobile Apps*: Developing apps that allow patients to engage in heartbeat meditation and track their emotional states can promote accessibility and adherence.
- *Telehealth*: Utilizing telehealth platforms to offer remote MHbT sessions can reach patients who may not have access to in-person therapy.

Promoting MHbT within community settings can foster greater awareness and understanding. Community workshops, support groups, and educational programs can introduce the principles of MHbT to individuals and families facing terminal illnesses.

In conclusion, the theoretical and practical foundations of Meditative Heartbeat Therapy (MHbT) provide a comprehensive framework for understanding its effectiveness in hospice and palliative care. By integrating concepts such as heartbeat awareness, emotional regulation, and the interconnectedness of mind and body, practitioners can create transformative experiences for patients and families.

As we continue to explore the multifaceted nature of MHbT, it is essential to remain open to the evolving landscape of healthcare. The potential for integration into diverse settings, along with the use of emerging technologies, will ensure that MHbT remains a vital tool in supporting emotional and spiritual well-being.

REFLECTION
EMBODYING THE RHYTHM OF LIFE

In moments of emotional upheaval—whether caused by grief, anxiety, or fear—there is often a yearning for stability, for something to hold on to. Meditative Heartbeat Therapy (MHbT) offers the heartbeat as this anchor. It is a rhythm that remains constant, even when everything else feels chaotic. The heartbeat teaches us that even in moments of inner turmoil, there is always something stable to return to.

This concept is at the heart of emotional regulation: the practice of coming back to the body when emotions become overwhelming. It is not about controlling what we feel or avoiding discomfort but learning to meet our emotions with presence and awareness. In MHbT, individuals are invited to anchor themselves to the rhythm of their heartbeat, using it as a compass to navigate emotional storms. With every beat, there is an opportunity to pause, breathe, and gently remind oneself: I am here. I am alive. I can sit with this.

This is the essence of emotional regulation through MHbT—not forcing emotions into submission but creating space for them to exist without overpowering us. When we connect with the heartbeat, we discover that emotions, like rhythms, rise and fall. They are not permanent states but waves that come and go. The heartbeat becomes a reminder that we are more than our emotional states; we are the steady rhythm beneath them.

Interoception: Listening to the Body's Messages

Interoception—the ability to sense and interpret internal bodily signals—plays a crucial role in how we understand and regulate our emotions. Many of us live disconnected from our bodies, unaware of the subtle signals that alert us to emotional shifts. Yet, these signals are always present, quietly guiding us. The heartbeat is one such signal—a continuous, reliable messenger.

Through MHbT, individuals develop their interoceptive awareness by tuning into the rhythm of their heart. As they listen, they begin to notice patterns: the way their heartbeat speeds up in moments of anxiety, slows during relaxation, or pulses gently in moments of sadness. This awareness becomes a powerful tool for emotional regulation, offering insight into how emotions manifest physically. With practice, individuals learn to respond to these signals with curiosity rather than judgment.

This connection between mind and body fosters a sense of agency. Instead of feeling overwhelmed by emotions, individuals learn to work with their bodies, using the heartbeat as a grounding tool. The body becomes an ally in emotional regulation rather than an obstacle to be overcome.

The practice of heartbeat awareness challenges the mind-body divide, inviting us to experience ourselves as fully embodied beings. There is often a tendency to prioritize thought over sensation, mind over body. Yet, MHbT reminds us that cognition is not something that happens solely in the brain—it is deeply rooted in the body.

When we listen to our heartbeat, we engage with the body not as a passive vessel but as an active participant in our emotional and cognitive experiences. The body holds memories, emotions, and knowledge that the mind alone cannot access. In MHbT, individuals learn to trust the wisdom of their bodies, discovering that their heartbeat can guide them toward emotional clarity and insight.

This embodied approach fosters a new way of being in the world —one that emphasizes presence, acceptance, and connection. It teaches us to move beyond the abstract and into the tangible, to live not only in our thoughts but in the felt experience of the body. As individuals engage with their heartbeat, they reconnect with a deeper sense of self—one that is grounded, whole, and fully alive.

Each heartbeat tells a story. It reflects not only our physical state but our emotional and inner journey. In MHbT, the heartbeat becomes a mirror—revealing patterns, insights, and truths that might otherwise remain hidden. Individuals may discover that their heartbeat quickens in the presence of certain memories or slows during moments of acceptance. These rhythms offer valuable insights into their emotional landscape.

Through this reflective practice, individuals begin to understand that their heartbeat is not something to be controlled but something to be listened to. It becomes a guide for self-inquiry, helping them explore questions such as: What does my heartbeat tell me about how I am feeling? What memories or emotions surface when I sit with this rhythm? In these moments of inquiry, the heartbeat becomes a gateway to deeper understanding.

This self-reflection is not always comfortable. It may bring unresolved emotions to the surface—grief, fear, regret. Yet, MHbT teaches that these emotions are not enemies to be defeated but messages to be received. They offer an opportunity for healing and reconciliation, for making peace with the past and embracing the present.

One of the key mechanisms explored in Chapter 2 is cognitive reappraisal—the ability to reinterpret a situation in a way that changes its emotional impact. MHbT offers a unique pathway to cognitive reappraisal through the simple act of heartbeat awareness. When individuals focus on their heartbeat, they engage in a process of reinterpretation—shifting their attention from fear to presence, from anxiety to acceptance.

For example, a person may initially experience fear while listening to their heartbeat, interpreting it as a reminder of life's fragility. Yet, through practice, they may come to see the same rhythm as a symbol of life's continuity—a comforting presence that connects them to their journey. This shift in perspective transforms the emotional experience, turning fear into acceptance and anxiety into peace.

This practice of reappraisal is not about denying difficult emotions but about meeting them with a new lens. It teaches individuals that their emotional responses are not fixed but fluid—that with awareness, they can change the way they relate to their experiences.

Beyond its psychological benefits, MHbT also offers a pathway to deeper reflection. The heartbeat serves as a reminder of the interconnectedness of all life—a rhythm that links the individual to the collective, the physical to the intangible. Many describe the experience of listening to their heartbeat as one of profound connection—both to themselves and to something greater.

In these moments, the heartbeat becomes more than a biological function; it becomes a symbol of presence and continuity. It invites individuals to explore questions of meaning, purpose, and connection. What does it mean to be alive? What legacy do I wish to leave behind? How can I find peace within this rhythm? These questions are not easily answered, but the heartbeat offers a space in which they can be explored.

In a world that often values productivity and efficiency, MHbT offers a radical invitation: to slow down, to listen, to be present. The practice of heartbeat awareness shifts our relationship with time. It teaches us that healing is not something that happens quickly but something that unfolds in the rhythm of presence.

This shift in perspective is particularly powerful for those facing the end of life. As they engage with their heartbeat, they learn to savor each moment, to find beauty in the ordinary, and to embrace the gift of presence. This practice offers a way of living that is not focused on the future or the past but grounded in the here and now.

Caregivers, too, benefit from this shift in perspective. By practicing MHbT alongside those they care for, they learn to be fully present—not only for others but for themselves. In these moments of shared presence, healing becomes a collective experience—a rhythm that unites us all.

As we move from the theoretical foundations of MHbT into its practical applications, let us carry forward the lessons of the heart-beat. Let us listen not only to our own rhythms but to the rhythms of those around us. Let us embrace the wisdom of the body, trusting that healing is not something we must force but something that unfolds naturally when we create space for it.

The heartbeat reminds us that we are never alone—that even in the midst of uncertainty, there is always a rhythm to guide us. Take a moment to place your hand over your chest. Feel the rhythm of your heart, and let it remind you: I am here. I am alive. I can sit with this.

PART TWO
SPIRITUAL, ETHICAL, AND PHILOSOPHICAL FOUNDATIONS

As the body begins to release and the breath becomes shallow, something profound unfolds—a return not only to silence, but to source. In this final section, we draw upon theological imagination, ecological spirituality, and embodied wisdom to offer a deeper framework for understanding MHbT as a sacred act. The chapters here explore the spiritual ecology of the cardiopulmonary system, the symbolic relationship between breath and soul, and the resonance of the heartbeat as a final liturgy. This is not an end, but an unveiling: a reminder that the spiritual body and the clinical body are never truly separate. Through sound, stillness, and sacred presence, MHbT becomes not only a therapy, but a theology—a way of seeing, of serving, and of surrendering.

CHAPTER 4

THE SPIRITUAL FOUNDATIONS OF MEDITATIVE HEARTBEAT THERAPY

No therapy is neutral. Every clinical gesture emerges from a worldview—often implicit, but always present. In MHbT, we begin by naming ours. This chapter explores the spiritual architecture upon which the practice rests: a framework that draws from dualism, panentheism, and a reverence for embodied transcendence. To understand the heartbeat as sacred is to first ask: What is the soul? And where does it dwell?

In the silent sanctum of our chest, the heartbeat persists—unseen, often unnoticed, yet ever faithful. It is the first sound we hear in the womb and the last to leave us at death. Between those two sacred thresholds, it holds rhythm to everything we know of life. In Meditative Heartbeat Therapy (MHbT), the heartbeat is not merely a biological function but a metaphysical bridge, a unifier of opposites —flesh and spirit, time and eternity, self and cosmos.

The spiritual foundation of MHbT lies in its recognition of the heartbeat as the site of integration between body and soul. It is where duality ceases. Here, in this rhythmic center, we find the paradox of human life: we are both creature and creator, bound by flesh and lifted by spirit. This chapter explores that paradox.

We will consider how the heartbeat transcends the Cartesian

divide, how it grounds the soul in the body and permits the divine to echo through our veins. Drawing from philosophy, cross-cultural mysticism, and clinical experience, we will trace the heartbeat as the sacred signature of life—a universal sign of the divine dwelling within the physical.

CARTESIAN DUALISM AND
THE HEART AS A LIMINAL ORGAN

René Descartes famously divided reality into *res extensa* (extended substance) and *res cogitans* (thinking substance). In this framework, the human being exists as a bifurcated entity: body and mind, matter and soul. The mystery of their union was, for Descartes, resolved by positing the pineal gland as the interface of body and soul. Yet this anatomical candidate never held the symbolic resonance of the heart.

In MHbT, the heartbeat—not the brain—is understood as the *living bridge* between these realms. It is at once purely physical—pumping blood, regulated by pacemaker cells—and yet profoundly spiritual: a rhythm that responds to love, grief, awe, fear, and tran-scendence. The heartbeat shifts when we see our beloved, when we weep, when we pray. It responds not merely to physiological inputs but to meaning itself

The heart, then, is not just an organ but a *liminal space*: the threshold where soul and flesh meet, touch, and become one.

A PHENOMENOLOGY OF THE HEARTBEAT:
EMBODIMENT AND DIVINITY

Phenomenology, particularly the work of Merleau-Ponty, teaches us that the body is not an object we possess but the very condition of our perception. We live through the body, and the heartbeat is the primal rhythm of that living. In MHbT, patients are invited to return to this fundamental rhythm, to listen not as an observer but as a participant in their own becoming.

The *experience* of the heartbeat during meditation reveals its dual nature: it anchors the self in the here-and-now while simultaneously opening a portal to the beyond. Patients often describe feeling "suspended between worlds," "floating in light," or "returning home." These are not mere poetic flourishes; they are authentic spiritual experiences rooted in the *felt sense* of the heart. To listen to the heartbeat is to return to the sacred center—to the place where life and consciousness first met.

In nearly every spiritual tradition, rhythm is divine. From the *aum* of the Upanishads to the Sufi whirling dervish, from Gregorian chant to Lakota drum circles, sacred sound marks the presence of the holy. The heartbeat—our first rhythm—stands among these as the most intimate of sacred sounds.

- *In Hinduism*, the cosmic sound *AUM* is said to be the primordial vibration from which all things arise. The heartbeat, echoing this vibration, is the personal *nada*, the inner sound of life.
- *In Sufi Islam*, the beating of the heart during *zikr* (remembrance of God) is a sacred practice, aligning the seeker with divine presence through rhythmic breath and movement.
- *In early Christianity*, desert mystics practiced *hesychasm*— the prayer of the heart—believing that through repetition of the Jesus Prayer, the physical heart could awaken to the indwelling Spirit
- *In Indigenous cosmologies*, especially among the Navajo and Andean peoples, the heartbeat of the Earth (often perceived through drumbeat or ceremony) is mirrored in the human heart. To live in rhythm with this beat is to live in harmony with the divine order of the world

MHbT carries forward this lineage by allowing the heartbeat to become a living prayer—a sound that is both physiological and metaphysical, personal and universal.

Over years of facilitating MHbT in hospice settings, patients and families have shared experiences that defy reduction to neurology alone. One woman, diagnosed with metastatic ovarian cancer, described the sound of her own heart as "a knocking from heaven." As her sessions continued, she began to visualize a glowing figure accompanying her, pulsing in time with her heartbeat.

Another patient—a former rabbi—spoke of hearing his father's voice within his own pulse. "I thought he was gone," he whispered, "but then I realized... he's inside me. I carry his rhythm."

These are not hallucinations. They are sacred perceptions. The dying often approach what Carl Jung called the *numinous*: experiences imbued with mystery, awe, and spiritual power. MHbT creates a container for these moments, allowing the patient to traverse the veil between body and soul without fear.

When the heart stops beating, the body ceases to circulate blood, and life—as we define it biologically—ends. But in MHbT, this moment is seen not as obliteration, but as *disentanglement*. It is the moment the soul, no longer tethered to the material rhythm of life, begins its own journey.

As long as the heartbeat continues, the soul and body are united —not fused, but interwoven. The heart's rhythm is the shared language of their union. It is *through* the heartbeat that the divine lives within the body. When that rhythm ends, the divine does not cease. It continues—freed from form.

For those present at the bedside, the silence that follows the final beat is often overwhelming. But for many MHbT practitioners, that silence is not empty. It is *threshold*—a sacred hush. Something has departed, not vanished.

MHbT does not end with the patient's death. Many families choose to keep the recording of their loved one's heartbeat as a sacred relic. Some play it during anniversaries, others integrate it into rituals of remembrance. These recordings become a *living echo*—proof that love continues to pulse in memory and presence.

One daughter, grieving the loss of her mother, described listening to the heartbeat recording every night before bed. "It's not about pretending she's still alive," she said. "It's about remembering that her rhythm shaped mine. I came into being listening to her heart. It's the sound I trusted before I had words."

In grief, the heartbeat becomes a bridge—not just between body and soul, but between *past and present, presence and absence.*

MHbT's metaphysical claim is simple, yet profound: every being with a heartbeat is both physical and divine. This applies not only to humans, but to all animals, even certain plants and invertebrates that maintain rhythmic circulatory pulses.

The implication is radical: all living beings are spiritual beings. The heartbeat is not exclusive to humans, and so divinity is not exclusive to humans either. We are all animated by the same sacred rhythm, pulsing from the same source.

This echoes the teachings of Indigenous traditions that speak of "All My Relations"—the belief that humans, animals, trees, rivers, and stars are kin. When we meditate on the heartbeat, we are not only entering communion with ourselves but with the entire web of life.

In mystic theology, the soul is said to carry a memory of its origin —a memory of union with the Divine. The heartbeat, in MHbT, becomes the *reverberation of that memory.* Each beat is a whisper: *You are of God. You are never separate.*

Patients sometimes report spontaneous tears during heartbeat meditation. "I don't know why I'm crying," they say. But the soul does. The body remembers its sacred origin. The tears are recognition.

As the philosopher Plotinus wrote, "We are not strangers here. We are exiles. But we remember." The heartbeat is the messenger of that remembrance. Its rhythm is a call to return—not to a place, but to a state of being.

The final gift of the heartbeat is that it teaches us how to *let go.* We do not beat our hearts by will; they beat through us. To trust the heartbeat is to trust life itself. This is the deepest practice of MHbT: learning to *die into the heart*—to surrender the need for control, to follow the rhythm to its final note.

Many dying individuals report that the most peace they've ever felt came in their final weeks—during sessions of simply listening to their own heart. In a culture obsessed with achievement and fear of death, MHbT offers a counteroffering: presence, rhythm, return.

In MHbT, the heartbeat is not a metaphor. It is a *revelation*. It reveals the unity of opposites: physical and spiritual, temporal and eternal. It shows us that while body and soul may be distinct, in life they are one—and that unity is made possible by the humble miracle of the heart.

When we listen to our heartbeat in meditation, we are listening to more than a muscle. We are listening to the divine signature of our existence. We are listening to the rhythm by which the soul made its home in the body—and through which it may one day return.

REFLECTION

ONE RHYTHM, ONE LIFE—
A MEDITATION ON THE SACRED HEARTBEAT

"We are not human beings having a spiritual experience.
We are spiritual beings having a human experience."
—Pierre Teilhard de Chardin

In the hush of a hospice room, long after the last breath has passed, silence does not feel empty. It feels full. Full of memory, of presence, of a rhythm that once was. A rhythm that still echoes.

That rhythm—our heartbeat—is the first sound of our life and, for those who love us, the last part of us they may remember with awe. We often forget it while we are alive. It slips into the background like the hum of a gentle tide. Yet it is this rhythm that carried us through every fear, every joy, every sacred moment of this life.

And perhaps more than anything else, it is this heartbeat that reveals the truth: we are not separate. Not from one another. Not from the world. Not from the Divine.

We begin in water, cradled in a womb. Long before we breathe, we listen. And what we hear is rhythm. A maternal pulse, steady and surrounding. It is our first intimacy, our first truth. We are born into rhythm, and we never leave it.

Even when we forget, the heart does not. It does not ask for our awareness. It beats in our joy and in our sorrow, in our sleep and in our waking. It beats when we are brokenhearted and when we are in love. It beats in prayer and in panic. It carries us forward, unwavering.

In a sense, this heartbeat is not the gift of a distant deity. It is the presence of the holy within the body. It is the evidence of Spirit made manifest in flesh.

We do not earn it. We do not control it. We inherit it, moment by moment. It reminds us that we belong to life.

Tradition teaches us that revelation is not sealed. Truth unfolds continuously—in science, in relationship, in lived experience. MHbT invites us to consider that perhaps the most constant revelation is one we carry within: the sound of our own heart. To listen to it is to practice reverence. It is to say: "Here I am. I am alive. This moment matters."

In MHbT, we teach patients and caregivers alike to pause. To place a hand on the chest. To feel the temple beneath their ribs. And to listen—not for answers, but for presence.

This act of listening is a kind of prayer. It does not require belief. It only requires attention. It says: "What is here matters. What is here is holy."

MHbT does not tell us what to believe. It simply gives us a place to listen.

If God is love, then the heartbeat is the drum of that love. If God is mystery, then the heartbeat is a gentle knocking from the unknown. If God is process, unfolding and unfinished, then the heartbeat is the tempo of our becoming.

No matter the theology, the message is the same: the heartbeat speaks. It speaks to our living. It speaks through our dying. It speaks even in absence.

After a death, the silence of a no-longer-beating heart can be almost unbearable. But even that silence is not void. It echoes. It reverberates in memory.

Families who have practiced MHbT often return to the recordings. Not to pretend their loved one is still here—but to remember that love, once given, is never lost. That rhythm lived in them. It still shapes them.

This is grief through the lens of reverence. This is remembrance not as clinging, but as celebration. We are made by the hearts of those we love. And even when they stop, something remains.

Some faiths affirm the interconnected web of existence. What better metaphor for that web than the shared rhythm of life

The heartbeat is not just human. It beats in the whale beneath the sea, in the deer in the forest, in the child yet unborn. It beats in every creature who has ever longed, loved, or leapt in joy.

To honor the heartbeat is to honor the whole. It is to remember that we are not above the world but within it. That we are not its masters, but its kin.

When we sit in MHbT and hear our heart, we do not only hear ourselves. We hear the rhythm of the cosmos playing through our ribs.

When death draws near, many patients describe a letting go—not in fear, but in grace. The body becomes still, and yet the heart remains for a while. It does not rush to leave.

In MHbT, we sit with that still-beating heart as long as it offers itself. We honor it. We say goodbye not only to a body but to a rhythm. A rhythm that carried a soul through the wild beauty of life.

There is no need for fear when we have already practiced this listening. We have already learned to trust the rhythm. We have learned to let it lead us. And when it stops, we let it go—not into void, but into mystery.

What will remain of us when we are gone? Our words may fade. Our images may blur. But our heartbeat—metaphorically or literally —will remain in those we touched.

Every person we loved, every hand we held, every child we rocked to sleep—they carry our rhythm.

This is the heart's great legacy: to be remembered not for what it achieved, but for how it was present. For how it pulsed gently through the world, beating alongside others.

This gospel: not that we are saved by faith, but that we are shaped by presence. That the holy is not beyond us, but within us. And it beats. And it beats. And it beats.

Now, place your hand over your chest. Breathe. Listen.

What you hear is not only the beat of your own body.

It is the rhythm of ancestors. The music of the cosmos. The whisper of Spirit.

It is your mother's heartbeat, which you once heard from within.

It is your child's heartbeat, which you once cradled in the crook of your arm.

It is your beloved's heartbeat, which you once listened to in the quiet of night.

And it is your own—faithful, enduring, present.

Let it teach you how to live.

Let it show you how to love.

And when the time comes, let it lead you home.

CHAPTER 5

THE BREATH OF THE SOUL

We have spoken of rhythm. Now we must speak of respiration. This chapter expands the conversation by drawing attention to the cardiopulmonary system as a unified ecology—one that nourishes not only the body, but the soul. Here, MHbT reaches into deeper terrain: the interbeing of breath and beat, of heart and lungs, of forest and body. What if the lungs were the stomach of the soul? What if each heartbeat was the echo of divine presence?

THE SILENT DANCE OF BREATH AND HEART

In the hushed light of dawn, I sit by her bedside, listening to the gentle rise and fall of her chest. Each inhale and exhale is a quiet promise, each heartbeat a steady drum in the silence. The candle on the nightstand flickers as if in time with this living music. Here at the edge of life, heart and lungs move together in an intimate pas de deux —the breath and the heartbeat entwined like lovers in a final dance. In these moments, the rhythm of her breath feels like a prayer, and her heartbeat like a hymn. The very air she inhales is itself a kind of communion, a gift from the world beyond these four walls. Her body is an ecosystem: lungs absorbing the world's breath, the heart pumping soul-enriched blood through her veins. This is the cardiopulmonary ecology—a sacred network of wind and flame, tide and pulse, that carries the human spirit.

Out in nature, we see that trees breathe carbon dioxide and give back oxygen; similarly, our lungs draw in life-giving air while our hearts consume it into purpose and being. In Greek myth, Gaia breathed life into man; in science, we know each breath refreshes our blood with oxygen to feed every cell. But at the bedside, these processes feel less mechanical and more mystical—the breath a direct thread to spirit, the heartbeat an echo of love. The heart and lungs here are like a river meeting the sea: one endless flow supporting the other. Each breath fosters the flame of life in her heart; each heartbeat fans the spark of life in her lungs. Together they compose a final serenade, an ecology of flesh and spirit, wind and warmth.

In palliative and hospice care, we learn to honor these rhythms. The supplemental oxygen humming softly at the bedside is more than a machine—it is a companion in this dance. As one hospice nurse once said to me, placing a gentle hand on the patient's chest, "Your breath is your prayer, and your heart carries that prayer to the sky." In Meditative Heartbeat Therapy (MHbT), we believe the breath and heartbeat are the vessels of the soul. They are the doorways through which spirit enters and leaves the body. To care for breath is to minister to spirit; to calm the heartbeat is to soothe the soul. In this chapter we explore how heart and lungs engage in this sacred partnership at the end of life, how clinicians and caregivers can tend to this inner ecosystem with both science and reverence, and how MHbT weaves together the physiological and the metaphysical into one tapestry of care.

"God breathed into Adam the breath of life," says Genesis; with one exhalation of the Creator, humankind became a living soul. Throughout the world's faiths, breath is synonymous with spirit. In Hebrew, *ruach* means both wind and spirit; in Greek *pneuma*, in Sanskrit *prāṇa*, in Latin *spiritus*—all tie the airy wind to the very essence of life. The Upanishads call breath the cosmic fire of creation. The Buddha instructed disciples to watch the breath (*ānāpā-nasati*) as the gateway to enlightenment. Indigenous elders pray with deep inhales and exhales, believing each breath draws in the Great Mystery. Even Mary Oliver reminded us that air is "our sweet necessity," a gift feeding *bone and soul* alike.

Likewise, the heart carries deep spiritual symbolism. In Christianity the heart is the seat of love and the indwelling of the Holy Spirit ("a new heart I will give you," said Ezekiel). Desert fathers prescribed the *prayer of the heart*, for their flock, believing each heartbeat could invoke the divine. In the Eastern tradition, the Sanskrit *hridaya* (heart) and *prāṇa* (breath) are seen as twin lights; yogis direct breath (pranayama) toward the heart-chakra, igniting a connection to higher consciousness. The Yoruba acknowledge Ẹ́dá (breath) and Ọkàn (heart) in healing rituals, seeing them as two faces of life. North American Indigenous peoples speak of the heart-lung as a single Lodge in the body—to breathe with a steady heart is to live in harmony with the world. Across faiths, breath is prayer, heartbeat is song.

In one Lakota prayer, it is said that "mitakuye oyasin"—"all beings[are] my relations"—for we all share this breath. An inhalation of one person is shared among all life, and each heartbeat resonates with the pulse of the cosmos. In each Christian or Muslim last rites ceremony, the family surrounds the dying, head bowed, whispering prayers with each slow breath of their loved one. Buddhists light incense and recite mantras in rhythm with the patient's pulse. These rites are not mere ritual; they are attempts to guide the sacred breath and heartbeat home. We find that when we consciously align our breathing with the pulse, body and soul seem to harmonize. The beating heart becomes a personal mantra. The traveling breath becomes like fire—the same element that fed the flame of creation now kindles our final journey.

Just as the Psalmist exhorts, *"Let everything that has breath praise the Lord,"* our lungs do as commanded, even in fragility. When we breathe, we inhale divinity; when our heart beats, it reminds us we are touched by the divine. This chapter does not exalt one tradition alone, but listens to these many voices—Christian hymn and Navajo lullaby, Vedic mantra and Jewish wind-song—all attesting to a simple truth: the breath of life and the rhythm of love are one. They are each other's keepers.

Beneath the layers of metaphor, the heart and lungs perform a marvel of physiology. It's a closed-loop ecosystem inside us. With each gentle breath, the lungs fill with air—oxygen enters tiny alveoli (air sacs) and passes into the blood. That blood, red and rich, flows into the left side of the heart, which then pumps it in a continuous circuit to every tissue. There, oxygen is delivered to cells, and carbon dioxide (the waste) is picked up. This deoxygenated blood returns to the right side of the heart, which sends it to the lungs once more. In essence, every inhalation and exhalation, every heartbeat and pause, is a turn of the ecological wheel of life.

Imagine a pair of partners in a dance: the lungs and the heart. One inhales and receives the world's breath; the other presses and propels that breath through the body. The lungs act as the earth's lungs—pulling in oxygen that plants have given forth and releasing carbon dioxide that will grow new forests. In our bodies, the heart is like a river's current, distributing nutrients (including oxygen) throughout the land of the body. If one partner falters, the dance stumbles. For example, when chronic obstructive pulmonary disease (COPD) robs the lungs of capacity, the heart must strain, pushing harder to circulate a sparser supply of oxygen. When the heart weakens in congestive failure, fluid may back up into the lungs (pulmonary edema), making breathing feel like wading through mud. This interdependence means that in hospice care, we rarely see problems of "just the heart" or "just the lungs"—they are forever intertwined.

Respiratory Sinus Arrhythmia: Even at rest, our breathing and heartbeat converse. You may not realize it, but with each inhale the heart briefly speeds up, and with each exhale it slows—a built-in mechanism called respiratory sinus arrhythmia. It is nature's way of optimizing gas exchange: during the inhale, our blood fills with oxygen so the heart can hurry it along; during the exhale, slowing the heart reduces unnecessary pumping, conserving energy. MHbT leverages this subtle conversation. By consciously lengthening the exhale to be twice as long as the inhale, for instance, one can magnify the heart's natural rhythm towards a calmer steadiness. In this sense, the breath is not only a vessel for life's gases but a lever on the heart's own tempo.

Chemical Dialogues: Deep in the brain, chemoreceptors monitor oxygen and carbon dioxide levels. When carbon dioxide rises, these receptors urge faster breathing; if oxygen dips, they whisper anxiety to hasten the heart. At the end of life, as these balances shift, patients often feel a panic in each breath, a wildfire of fear stoked by unmet gas exchange. As caregivers, we remember that the flaring anxiety over shortness of breath is physiological as much as existential. When oxygen is scarce, the body sounds alarms. This is why oxygen therapy is so central in hospice—a gift of ease for those whose lungs are fatigued. Yet we also understand it is more than a treatment; it is a symbol of care, an intervention that, in MHbT practice, can be baptized with meaning.

Ecological Metaphors: In the rainforest of our body, lungs are the leaves of the great tree, capturing the sun's breath (oxygen) and giving life to every limb (the body's tissues). The heart is the river irrigating that tree, ensuring the leaves stay green and the roots firm. Consider the ocean and sky: we breathe the same oceanic oxygen as whales do, and our hearts pump that shared blessing. The blood in your veins is the same saltwater of life that once surrounded dinosaurs, that still roars in every throat. Each heartbeat sends micro-volcanoes of life through your body—a scintillating pulse of energy recycled from starlight and wind. When we unite the breath and heart through MHbT, we are acknowledging that inner forest, river, and sky. We sit with the patient in the temple of their own nature.

CASE EXAMPLE: MIGUEL'S STORY

Miguel is a 67-year-old retired carpenter with advanced COPD from a lifetime of smoking. His lungs have become rigid and hollowed, like old bellows barely inflating. At hospice entry he was on 4L/min of supplemental oxygen via nasal cannula. His wife describes him as "afraid of each new breath." Indeed, Miguel often sat hunched in his favorite recliner, needles of anxiety shooting into his chest every time he gasped for air. His heart would race to compensate, and he would worry the next heartbeat was his last.

When I first met him, I placed a hand over his heart and taught him to place another over his belly. "Feel these two beats," I said. "Every breath, your heart beats — they are companions." We practiced a slow, even breathing: four seconds inhale, hold two, eight seconds exhale through pursed lips. With my watch, we counted softly. We synchronized the long exhale with his heart's slowing. At first he laughed, "I never thought of breathing as something to do!" But by the third minute, his pulse had steadied, his forehead smoothed.

OVER DAYS, MHbT became part of Miguel's routine. He would sit by the window each morning, eyes closed, hands resting in his lap. We would play a quiet recording of his own heartbeat (from a digital stethoscope), a rich thrum he now recognized as his own life-song. As he listened, I guided him to breathe in harmony with that rhythm. Inhaling to the beat, and exhaling on its soft fade, he described feeling "centered in a way pills never gave." His oxygen saturation, usually bouncing in the low 80s, would inch into the low 90s during our sessions—a quiet testament that calm breathing really did help blood flow.

Spiritually, Miguel, raised a Buddhist, began to speak in gentle awe about feeling connected to something greater. "I can't see it," he said one afternoon, tears in his eyes, "but I feel a light through this

sound [of his heartbeat] and breath, like we're all the same breath."
His wife held his hand and whispered the *Om mani padme hum*,
combining her Christian rosary with his mantras. Together in silence,
they created a sacred space around his chairs, an altar of heart and
breath. In four weeks, Miguel's anxiety attacks faded; he eventually
even asked to be alone at night without his wife touching his oxygen
mask, saying he could "hold the machine in my mind now, like it's
glowing."

Miguel's case shows the ecology at work: as we nurtured his
breathing, his heart relaxed; as we grounded his heart, his breath
calmed. His own breath became a ritual of peace and connection, a
final prayer of love in each inhale.

BREATHING WITH THE HEART:
ENTRAINMENT AND TECHNIQUE

In MHbT we speak of *entrainment*—the practice of bringing the
breath and heartbeat into a shared rhythm. Just as a choir can sing in
harmony once the choir master sets the pace, we help patients find a
tempo where breathing and pulse gently synchronize. This shared
tempo can be summoned with intention:

1. *Play the Beat:* Gently lay a hand on your chest or have a
   caregiver place their hand lightly on the patient's heart.
   Turn on the recording of the patient's heartbeat and listen
   to the steady, reliable beat. Let your attention rest on this
   rhythm as an anchor.
2. *Steady Inhalation:* Breathe in slowly through the nose on a
   quiet count (for example, to the count of three or four),
   feeling the lungs expand and the abdomen rise. Try to
   draw the inhale in time with your heartbeat—if
   comfortable, breathe in on every second or third beat, as
   guided.
3. *Gentle Exhalation:* Exhale fully through gently pursed lips,
   doubling the time of your inhale if you can (perhaps to a

count of six or eight). Many patients find it calming to exhale on the heart's slow, retreating beat. Notice your heart slowing slightly as you release each breath.

4. *Pause and Listen:* After exhaling, allow a brief natural pause before the next breath. In this space, simply listen to the pulse and enjoy the quiet between breaths.

5. *Repeat with Intention:* Continue this cycle for several minutes. The goal is not to force, but to allow breath and heartbeat to inform each other—your lungs filling and emptying in a duet with your heart's cadence.

6. *Focus on Sensation:* Invite the patient (or practice yourself) to sense the warmth of blood under the palm, the gentle expansion of the chest, and even the subtle vibration of blood flow in quiet. Sometimes placing a hand on the belly and one on the chest helps track both breathing and heartbeat together.

7. *Visualization:* It may help to imagine the breath as a gentle tide, and the heartbeat as the shoreline: with each inhale, the waves (breath) push into the sand (heart), with each exhale, the waves recede, and the shore remains. Or envision the heart as a drum slowly echoing, and each breath is a quiet bell toll aligning with the rhythm.

8. *Positive Cueing:* Often we use compassionate words to nurture the practice: "With each breath, you are supported by the heartbeat of love," or "Your inhalation draws in courage; your exhale releases pain." Framing these actions as acts of love and presence keeps the patient engaged and calm.

When we speak of heart-lung entrainment, medical terms come into play—we slow the *respiratory rate* (the number of breaths per minute) and by prolonging each exhale, we boost *vagal tone*, encouraging the heart to rest. The gentle increase in oxygen saturation from slower, deeper breaths also feeds the tissues more efficiently, reducing shortness of breath. But alongside these metrics, we observe emotional shift: shoulders drop, eyes close in ease, color returns to flushed cheeks. The very act of co-regulating breath and beat can feel like an embrace between body and soul.

Throughout history, people intuitively practiced such techniques. Ancient yogis taught that a breath retained as long as the heartbeat would unite body and spirit (hence techniques like anulom-vilom or even simple belly breathing). The early Christian hermits prayed with Luke 1:37, "with God nothing shall be impossible," mentally aligning faith with breath. In reiki, life-force practitioners sometimes mirror the patient's inhale with their own exhale to transfer calm. In MHbT, we formalize these insights into a gentle practice.

CASE EXAMPLE: ANITA'S STORY

Anita, a 75-year-old retired nurse, suffered from end-stage congestive heart failure due to longstanding hypertension. Her swollen legs were testament to the heart's fatigue; her lungs crackled with fluid when examined. She required supplemental oxygen at 2L/min, but still complained of feeling like she was "drowning on dry land." Anita was a woman of deep Christian faith, and often recited the Lord's Prayer when distressed, pausing mid-breath as the tears flowed.

Working with Anita, I combined her own coping mechanisms with MHbT. I asked if we could try something together: she breathed in deeply as if inhaling the Lord's mercy; then, on one beat of her heart (felt under her palm), we both recited "... give us this day our daily bread." She exhaled quietly on "Amen," imagining it as if releasing a bouquet of incense to heaven. For Anita, each cycle of prayer and breath became an entrainment of the heart's devotion with the lungs' sustenance.

We also used practical breathing techniques: Anita learned *pursed-lip breathing*—inhaling through the nose, then exhaling slowly through pursed lips (as if blowing out a candle), to keep her airways open longer. Whenever she began to panic, I placed my hand gently on her chest and whispered, "Inhale on my heartbeat, let it steady us." Miraculously, her heart rate would respond, falling from the low

100s into the 70s over a few breaths, and her oxygen saturation would climb into the upper 90s. Her nurses noted the shift: where prior to MHbT sessions Anita's respirations hit 30/min, afterward they slowed to 18–20/min, and she spoke more of acceptance than of fear.

Anita's story shows how cultural and spiritual traditions can join with technique. Her familiarity with prayer allowed a seamless entry into a breathing practice. She even taught her grandchildren a version of it: "Close your eyes, place one hand on your heart, and breathe slowly with me while we thank God." In her final weeks, Anita reported that when her breathing became very shallow, she would silently continue the exercise "in my mind." On the day she passed, her family swore they heard her whisper "peace" in rhythm with her last breaths. The harmony of her heart and lungs gave her and her loved ones the gift of a peaceful transition.

THE ART OF CARE:
HOLISTIC CARDIOPULMONARY SUPPORT

Breathing and beating are not just physiological facts—they are the focus of our clinical caregiving. In hospice, we use many tools to support this cardiopulmonary sanctuary. Some are medical (pumps, oxygen machines, medications), and some are tender and human (hand on heart, the sound of a beloved's voice). Both realms matter deeply.

- *Supplemental Oxygen:* We will soon note how oxygen therapy can ease the work of breathing. In that chapter we will give it a name: "sacred companion." Each liter per minute is indeed a gift of ease. Practitioners adjust flows to maintain comfort: often they aim for an SpO_2 of around 92–95% in active distress, understanding that chasing 100% is neither achievable nor necessary. We perform humidification (to moisten the dried membranes), change tubing, and reposition cannulas to reduce discomfort. A nasal cannula can feel strange on dry nostrils. Each box-like concentrator or cylinder in the room is not just a machine, but a kind of guardian of breath. We reframe it so for ourselves and families. One patient termed the soft hiss of the concentrator a "mechanical lullaby," something we try to share: when the machine turns on with a quiet whine, I might softly say to the patient, "Listen, it is singing us a song of comfort." In this way, the clinician's attitude can transform the environment: the tubes become "gentle vines," the mask a "soft crown of safety."

- *Positioning and Comfort:* Elevating the head of the bed (semi-Fowler's position) is a simple yet profound aid. When flat, patients often feel suffocated; seated, gravity helps the diaphragm. We fold pillows behind the back, and prop legs up to reduce edema. A gentle fan or air-circulator aimed lightly at the face can physically ease dyspnea (cool air against the face can trigger a reflex that slows respiratory drive). We keep blankets light—too much warmth can breed restlessness. Each of these may seem ordinary tasks, but in MHbT we frame them with intention: "This pillow holds you, these pillows breathe with you, each a cloud of comfort."

- *Medication:* Intractable breathlessness is often treated with low-dose opioids (like morphine) to blunt the sensation of air hunger, and sometimes with anxiolytics for panic. We explain to families that these are not "clock-stopping drugs," but tools to ease the tide of air so that each breath can be more of a grateful sigh. We must chart carefully, too: notes might read, "Reduced tachypnea from 30 to 22 with low-dose morphine, patient reports calmer breathing." Yet each drug dose in MHbT is offered also with presence: a soft hand on the shoulder, a permission to let go. If a ventilator or BiPAP is in use, we honor it as best we can, but often in hospice the goal is withdrawal of aggressive measures in favor of comfort. When noninvasive ventilation is needed briefly, we will nevertheless use MHbT principles: if a mask is on, we may have the patient imagine the mask as "a gentle warrior's shield," guiding each breath inward.

- *Communication and Presence:* Perhaps the most powerful interventions are hands and words. Sitting near the patient, holding a chest, we may silently synchronize breaths. We often say minimal soothing phrases: "I'm here, steady with your breath," or we mirror their inhalation with our own exhale. Families are gently invited to join: "Place your hand here," we coach a daughter, "and breathe together, one long breath in on Mama's heartbeat." This shared breath can feel sacred—a son and mother linking life forces for a moment. At times, a chaplain may sing a lullaby, or recite a comforting mantra, their cadence aligning with the rhythm we set. A small wooden crucifix or prayer card on the table and the slow breath become intertwined in the patient's mind; in one case, a Jewish patient spoke of feeling "as if the Sh'ma was flowing in my veins with each breath" once we had guided him to quietly recite it on his exhale.
- *"Altar of Breath":* We often say that in every hospice room, there is an invisible circle gathered around one altar—the patient's own breath and heartbeat. The nurse, aide, chaplain, family, volunteer—all present in body or spirit —form a living sanctuary. Oxygen tubes may snake like soft vines to this altar, feeding its flame. In MHbT we mind this circle: we enter gently and sit down, never rush it, and we remind everyone that their presence is participation. Sometimes at shift change, the next nurse will place a comforting hand on the patient and say, "I know they are safe with me. I will breathe with them." This echo of care seals the continuity of the circle.
- *Frame End-of-Life Rituals:* As death nears, caregivers often incorporate specific rituals tied to breath. In some Catholic homes, anointing oil is breathed in as we speak

"Into your hands, Lord, I commend [Name]." We may have families gather and each exhale together when the patient takes their last breath, symbolically sharing their sorrow and release. A Maori patient's family chanted an ancestral welcome (karanga) in unison with his rhythmic breathing. In Interfaith environments, any such gesture becomes meaningful: the breath and beat are universal sacraments.

Case Example (continued): It was especially poignant to see the cardiopulmonary ecology at work when Miguel's family took part. His granddaughter, clutching a "lucky penny" to his chest, recited a children's rhyming prayer in Spanish each time he inhaled, "A breath for me, a breath for you." At one point, Miguel grasped the air around his nose with a focused intent and said, "I can feel the grace in this air." The room—with its concentrator humming, a small bowl of water at the bedside, a red geranium and a framed photo of his wedding—became a microcosm of life. In those moments, every nurse's charting note ("O2 set at 3L, calm breathing achieved") felt like a translation of a sacred script.

THE PULSE OF PRESENCE

In the ecology of the dying, heart and lungs are inseparable. They weave together body and soul in the most elemental human way. Through MHbT we honor that tapestry: we sit with the breath and heartbeat as we would with an infant cradle or a cherished lullaby. Every inhale is an echo of creation; every heartbeat, a vow of fidelity. To care for the breath is to care for the soul; to entrain the heart's rhythm with the breath is to find harmony in chaos.

Over the years, I have watched many souls pass gently when guided by these rhythms. I remember an old Cherokee healer who once said, "When the time comes, our ancestors breathe for us." In that tradition, breathing becomes a communal act—and truly, in MHbT, we become the patient's ancestors in spirit, breathing with them until the last.

The heart's final beat need not be a drum of fear but a final pulse of love. The last breath can be an offering—a calm extinguishing of candlelight. As one of our nurses put it while placing a hand on a chest, "One heartbeat, one breath, one word: love." We leave this bedside practice knowing that in honoring the breath and the heart, we honor life itself.

When we close the door behind us, that invisible circle remains— the candle still flickering, the tubes coiled at rest. We carry with us the knowledge that somewhere in the quiet room, the soul has taken flight on the wings of a breath, to the eternal heartbeat that binds us all.

REFLECTION
THE BODY'S LAST OFFERING

I have come to believe that dying is not a breaking, but a thinning—of walls, of veils, of breath. At the end, the body doesn't fight so much as it begins to give back: its breath to the trees, its rhythm to the silence, its warmth to the waiting air. I once sat with a man who had not spoken in days. His breath was shallow, held like a whisper on the edge of wind. A recorded heartbeat played softly beside him, and for a moment it seemed his chest rose in rhythm to its sound—not perfectly, but enough. His daughter leaned in and whispered, "He used to say his heart was a drum." And there it was—the breath still moving, the heart still echoing, even as the body dimmed.

In these moments, I do not see organs. I see altars. The lungs as vessels that once held the breath of laughter, of grief, of prayers no one heard but God. The heart as a steady witness to it all. What a gift, to have been animated by wind and pulse. What a blessing, to let that breath return to the trees and the sky, as quietly as it came. In MHbT, we do not resist this return—we honor it. We walk beside it with rhythm, with reverence, with deep listening. The soul knows the way. And the body, in its final offering, remembers how to sing it home.

CHAPTER 6
THE HEART AND THE BARDO

For most of my professional life, I have worked with individuals at the precipice of life and death. I have sat at countless bedsides, holding hands that grew colder with each passing moment, whispering words of comfort to the dying as they stood at the threshold of the unknown. I have seen eyes, once bright with life, begin to shift their gaze toward something unseen—toward a realm just beyond our ordinary senses. And I have heard, time and again, those in their final moments speak of visions, voices, and presences that seem to beckon them forward. These experiences, rich in mystery and meaning, led me to develop Meditative Heartbeat Therapy (MHbT). In addition to many other benefits, the practice offers a profound opportunity: a glimpse into the Bardo—the transitional state between life, death, and rebirth described in *The Tibetan Book of the Dead*.

The Bardo is not merely a metaphysical construct but a lived reality that I have witnessed unfold in my patients. Within the rhythmic meditations and heartbeat entrainment of MHbT, I have seen individuals touch the edge of something vast—whether one calls it the afterlife, the dream state of consciousness, or the liminal passage between worlds. This introduction will explore how MHbT serves as a bridge between the living and the dying, offering an experiential pathway into the mysteries of the Bardo.

The *Bardo Thodol*, or *The Tibetan Book of the Dead*, teaches that the period following death is not a singular moment of cessation but a process—a passage through various states of awareness. It speaks of luminous visions, terrifying deities, and the mirror of one's karma reflecting back in the form of hallucinations and apparitions. To the untrained mind, these experiences can be overwhelming, but to those prepared through meditative practice, the Bardo is a space of liberation. The core of this teaching is that consciousness does not end with death; rather, it transitions through different states of awareness before rebirth or release.

In my work, I have encountered patients who, through guided heartbeat meditation, have entered states of consciousness that parallel the descriptions found in *The Tibetan Book of the Dead*. They have reported seeing light, feeling themselves float outside their bodies, or even encountering figures from their past or mythological landscapes that align with Eastern descriptions of the post-mortem journey. This is not a matter of blind faith but a testament to the power of the human mind and spirit when given the right tools to explore the liminal spaces between life and death.

At the core of MHbT is the use of the heartbeat as an anchor—both to the body and beyond it. The practice involves synchronizing breath with the natural rhythm of the heart, creating a state of deep focus where awareness expands beyond ordinary perception. This rhythmic entrainment echoes the meditative techniques described in the Tibetan traditions, where the practitioner learns to dissolve their egoic self into the sound of sacred mantras or the visualization of celestial deities.

Several patients who have undergone MHbT have described sensations of dissolution, of their sense of self blurring at the edges, as though they were stepping beyond the confines of their own physical form. Some have recounted visions of tunnels of light, faces appearing from the shadows, and moments of profound peace as though they were suspended in a vast and boundless space. One particular case stands out vividly: a woman in her late sixties, living with advanced-stage pancreatic cancer, who described the sensation of floating above her body while listening to the rhythmic beat of her own heart. She spoke of a "great golden light" and a presence that seemed to welcome her, only for her awareness to return as the session ended. This experience bears striking resemblance to descriptions in *The Tibetan Book of the Dead*, where the initial phase of the Bardo presents a radiant luminosity that the soul may either embrace or shy away from.

Visualization exercises are integral to MHbT, and they serve a function remarkably similar to the Tibetan practice of *Phowa*, the transference of consciousness at the time of death. Through guided imagery, patients are led into landscapes that mirror the terrain of the Bardo—a space where the boundaries between self and other begin to dissolve. In Tibetan Buddhist practice, practitioners are trained to visualize peaceful and wrathful deities, preparing the mind to recognize these apparitions as projections of their own consciousness when death finally arrives.

MHbT patients have reported similar encounters, albeit through the lens of their own cultural and personal beliefs. A retired physicist undergoing MHbT sessions described seeing a "river of stars" that he felt compelled to cross. Another patient, a former artist, saw a mandala of shifting colors and forms, pulsating in time with her breath, a vision not unlike the luminous fields described in the *Bardo Thodol*. These experiences suggest that the mind, when liberated from the constraints of ordinary thought, may indeed touch upon realities beyond our immediate comprehension.

Skeptics might argue that these experiences are merely neurological phenomena, the result of hypoxia or the hallucinatory effects of the dying brain. However, I would argue that this reductionist approach fails to grasp the profundity of what is being witnessed. The lived experiences of patients, many of whom have no prior knowledge of Tibetan eschatology, align too closely with the descriptions in *The Tibetan Book of the Dead* to be dismissed as mere coincidence.

Furthermore, the therapeutic benefits of these experiences cannot be ignored. Those who have glimpsed these altered states often report a lessening of their fear of death. They approach their final days with a greater sense of peace, knowing that death is not an abrupt void but a process, a journey akin to birth. Some even express joy, a quiet excitement at the prospect of entering the next stage of being. The clinical implications of this are profound: if we can use MHbT to prepare individuals for death in a way that brings them comfort, we are not just easing suffering—we are transforming the very experience of dying.

Meditative Heartbeat Therapy is more than a practice; it is a way of seeing, a way of experiencing the profound mystery that surrounds us in every breath, every beat of the heart. Through rhythmic meditation and guided visualization, it offers a doorway into the Bardo, allowing individuals a glimpse of what lies beyond the veil of ordinary consciousness.

In a world that often seeks to deny death, MHbT stands as a radical assertion that death is not an end but a transition, an unfolding of consciousness into something greater. Whether one believes in reincarnation, the afterlife, or the dissolution of self into the vast cosmos, the experiences of those who have undergone MHbT suggest that something persists, something continues. And if we can learn to navigate this passage with awareness and grace, we may find that death is not to be feared, but embraced as the next great journey.

REFLECTION
THRESHOLDS, ECHOES,
AND THE UNFINISHED SONG

The Bardo is often described as a passage—a corridor between worlds. But to me, it has never felt like a hallway. It feels more like a shoreline. Some step quietly into the surf, water curling around their feet. Others are swept by a sudden wave, gasping, wide-eyed. And then there are those who pause—one foot in, one foot behind—listening to the sound of the tide, unsure if it is calling them forward or back.

I once sat beside a man, Julian, a retired engineer whose life had been governed by logic and precise measurement. In his final days, he was mostly nonverbal, but one evening he opened his eyes and whispered, "I think I'm between floors. Like in an elevator, but I can't tell if it's going up or down." He smiled faintly. "But I'm not afraid." The heartbeat track was playing gently beside him, and I remember thinking: *perhaps this is what the Bardo feels like—not a judgment, not a reckoning, but a weightless suspension.* A space between pulses.

There is something radically honest about this liminal state. The dying often become mystics—not by dogma, but by proximity. As clinicians, caregivers, and companions, we must learn to honor the Bardo not only as an esoteric concept, but as an observable, emotional, and spiritual reality. Meditative Heartbeat Therapy gives us a language and a ritual for this space. It allows us to sit in the silence between heartbeats and recognize it not as absence, but as sacred interval.

I've noticed that the dying begin to look toward corners more often. Their eyes drift to spaces that, to us, appear empty. They speak to people we cannot see. They reach for light that flickers outside our visible range. This is not confusion. This is awareness expanding. One woman said, "I'm not sure if I'm dreaming or dying, but the music is beautiful." And in that moment, I believed her. There was no chaos in her voice, no panic. Only music we could not hear.

If the heart is the soul's drum, then perhaps the Bardo is its echo —a reverberation of all that we've loved, feared, and carried. It is the space where the ego begins to loosen its grip, where the self dissolves into sensation, memory, and light. And MHbT, in its gentleness, helps people enter that echo with softness. It is not a pushing or a guiding —it is an accompaniment, a holding of space so that the soul may listen to itself one final time.

Sometimes, in MHbT sessions, patients begin to cry—not out of sadness, but relief. As if their bodies recognize something they've forgotten: the rhythm they were born into, the silence they will return to. One patient, moments before her final breath, whispered, "I can hear the rhythm of something larger than me. And it's not ending. I'm just joining it." I've never forgotten that. Not because it answered a question, but because it undid the need to ask.

The Bardo is not a place we must fully understand. It is not a hallway we must map. It is enough to know that it exists—and that it is not empty. Through MHbT, we sit beside those standing at its threshold, offering them the comfort of rhythm and the dignity of presence. We do not need to explain what comes next. We need only to listen with reverence, heartbeat to heartbeat, as they step into the unfinished song of what comes after.

CHAPTER 7

ETHICAL CONSIDERATIONS AND CHALLENGES IN IMPLEMENTING MHbT

In the realm of healthcare, ethical considerations are paramount, particularly when working with vulnerable populations such as patients in hospice and palliative care. Meditative Heartbeat Therapy (MHbT) presents unique ethical challenges that practitioners must navigate to ensure that the therapy is delivered safely, respectfully, and effectively.

This chapter explores the ethical principles that underpin MHbT, including autonomy, beneficence, non-maleficence, and justice. It also addresses cultural sensitivity, informed consent, and the importance of tailoring the therapy to meet the diverse needs of patients and families. Through careful consideration of these factors, practitioners can foster an environment of trust and collaboration, ultimately enhancing the therapeutic experience.

Autonomy is the ethical principle that emphasizes the right of individuals to make informed decisions about their own lives and healthcare. In the context of MHbT, it is essential to respect patients' autonomy by providing them with information about the therapy and allowing them to choose whether to engage in it.

Obtaining informed consent is a critical component of respecting patient autonomy. Practitioners should ensure that patients understand:

- The purpose of MHbT.
- The techniques involved in the therapy.
- Any potential risks or benefits associated with the practice.

When introducing MHbT to a new patient, a practitioner should explain the process in clear, accessible language. They might say, "We will record your heartbeat, and you'll listen to it as a way to help you relax and explore your feelings. Is this something you would like to try?" This open dialogue allows patients to make informed decisions about their participation.

The principles of *beneficence* and *non-maleficence* emphasize the obligation to act in the best interest of patients and to do no harm. Practitioners of MHbT should strive to create a safe and supportive environment where patients can explore their emotions without feeling overwhelmed or threatened.

Practitioners must be vigilant in assessing whether the emotional exploration encouraged by MHbT is appropriate for each individual. For some patients, engaging deeply with their emotions may trigger distressing feelings. In these cases, practitioners should prioritize the patient's well-being, offering support and adjusting the approach as necessary.

If a patient exhibits signs of acute distress during a session, the practitioner should pause the session and provide immediate emotional support. They might say, "I can see that this is difficult for you. Let's take a moment to breathe together and discuss how you're feeling."

The principle of *justice* pertains to fairness in the distribution of healthcare resources and the equitable treatment of all patients. In the context of MHbT, practitioners should ensure that the therapy is accessible to individuals from diverse backgrounds, including those from marginalized communities.

Practitioners should be mindful of cultural differences when implementing MHbT. This includes understanding how various cultural beliefs may influence a patient's perception of death, emotional expression, and therapeutic practices. And always remember to:

- Engage in open conversations about cultural preferences and beliefs during initial assessments.
- Adapt MHbT practices to align with patients' cultural backgrounds when possible.

CHALLENGES IN IMPLEMENTING MHBT

Implementing MHbT in healthcare settings may encounter logistical challenges, including time constraints, resource availability, and staff training.

In busy healthcare environments, practitioners often face limited time to conduct in-depth MHbT sessions. To address this, practitioners can:

- Offer brief, focused sessions (5–10 minutes) that can easily fit into patients' care routines.
- Create audio recordings of heartbeat meditations that patients can use independently between sessions.

Effective implementation of MHbT requires practitioners to be adequately trained in the techniques and principles underlying the therapy. However, there may be barriers to obtaining this training.

- Develop in-house training programs that provide hands-on experience with MHbT techniques.
- Utilize online resources, webinars, and workshops to educate staff on the practice.

Not all patients may feel ready to engage in MHbT, particularly if they are experiencing acute distress or emotional numbness. Practitioners must assess each patient's readiness for this type of emotional exploration. To encourage engagement, the practitioner may want to:

- Begin with introductory sessions that focus on relaxation techniques before delving into heartbeat awareness.
- Use supportive language to encourage patients to express their feelings and concerns about the therapy.

CULTURAL SENSITIVITY IN MHBT PRACTICE

Cultural beliefs and values significantly influence how patients perceive illness, death, and emotional expression. Practitioners must be aware of these cultural contexts when implementing MHbT.

Healthcare organizations should provide cultural competence training to staff, enabling them to:

- Recognize and respect diverse cultural perspectives.
- Adapt MHbT practices to align with patients' cultural beliefs and values.

Practitioners should be prepared to adapt MHbT to meet the needs of various cultural groups. This may involve incorporating cultural rituals or practices that resonate with patients. For example:

- For Indigenous patients, integrating drumming or storytelling elements can enhance the connection to MHbT.
- For patients with spiritual beliefs, incorporating prayers or affirmations during heartbeat meditation can foster a deeper sense of peace.

ETHICAL DILEMMAS IN MHBT

Practitioners may encounter ethical dilemmas that arise from conflicts of interest, such as the pressure to deliver certain therapies despite potential risks. Maintaining a focus on patient well-being is essential. Strategies for resolution may include:

- Engage in collaborative decision-making with patients and their families.
- Prioritize transparency, allowing patients to voice their concerns and preferences openly.

During MHbT sessions, practitioners may encounter patients who become overwhelmed by their emotions. It is vital to approach these situations with sensitivity. To respond to distress:

- Acknowledge the patient's feelings and create a safe space for expression.
- Offer grounding techniques or pause the session if necessary, allowing the patient to regain composure before continuing.

By focusing on autonomy, beneficence, non-maleficence, and justice, practitioners can deliver MHbT in a manner that is respectful, inclusive, and effective.

Addressing the challenges associated with MHbT requires collaboration, cultural sensitivity, and ongoing education. By prioritizing ethical practice, healthcare professionals can foster an environment where patients feel safe to explore their emotions, cultivate resilience, and find peace in their final days.

REFLECTION
THE HEARTBEAT AS A COMPASS
THROUGH LIFE'S GREATEST QUESTIONS

The heartbeat is a profound symbol, representing not only vitality and connection but also the impermanence of life. In the practice of Meditative Heartbeat Therapy (MHbT), we are invited to reflect on a truth that, while inevitable, is often difficult to face: our time in this world is finite. This awareness of life's fragility can evoke fear or sadness, but it also has the potential to awaken deep transformation, clarity, and meaning.

As we sit with the rhythm of our heartbeat, we are invited to confront the unknown—not as something to be feared, but as an essential part of the human journey. Each beat becomes a gentle reminder that life is a flow—an ongoing, ever-changing process. Through the practice of MHbT, we learn to ask: *What truly matters to me? What am I offering to the world, both now and in the future?* The heartbeat does not demand answers, but it invites us to look inward and find meaning in the present moment, where life's significance resides not in grand achievements or external validation, but in the small, intimate moments—moments of presence, connection, and love.

Listening to the heartbeat becomes a form of meditation that invites us to reconcile with life's impermanence. Just as the heart continues to beat without our conscious effort, life continues to unfold, regardless of our desire for control or certainty. This realization encourages us to release our grip on expectations, relinquishing the need to know every answer. In this openness, we find that the beauty of life lies not in certainty but in the willingness to embrace uncertainty, to live fully in the present without the burden of anticipating the future.

MHbT teaches us that life and death are not opposites, but two interconnected parts of the same cycle. Much like the contraction and expansion of the heart, life requires both holding on and letting go. We often experience this paradox in our own lives—joy and sorrow, hope and fear, connection and loss—yet in many cultures, there is an inclination to avoid or suppress the presence of death and suffering. However, MHbT shows us that life's most profound wisdom comes not from resisting or evading death, but from holding both life and death in our awareness simultaneously.

Each heartbeat symbolizes the rhythm of beginnings and endings, arrivals and departures. By tuning into this heartbeat, we are invited to sit with the discomfort of uncertainty and loss, but also to recognize that death is not a final end. It is a continuation of life's natural rhythm. In MHbT, patients learn that they do not need to solve the mystery of death or eliminate suffering in their lives. Instead, they are encouraged to meet each moment as it is— embracing both the grief and the gratitude, the fear and the peace, the sorrow and the joy.

For caregivers, this understanding is equally transformative. They are invited to move beyond the impulse to "fix" every situation and instead approach the complexity of care with open-hearted presence. In learning to hold space for both joy and sorrow, caregivers can cultivate a deeper sense of compassion, not just for those they care for, but also for themselves.

One of the most powerful aspects of MHbT is its capacity to facilitate emotional healing, particularly through forgiveness. The practice of tuning into the heartbeat provides space for unresolved emotions to surface—emotions that may have been buried or left unspoken.

These emotions may include old resentments, regrets, or the pain of unfinished conversations. The quiet space of heartbeat meditation allows for these emotions to emerge, not for analysis or judgment, but simply for presence and acceptance.

Forgiveness, in this context, is not an immediate action or a decision to let go, but a process—a gentle opening of the heart. Through the deep listening that MHbT encourages, we begin to understand that forgiveness is less about absolving others or erasing past wrongs, and more about freeing ourselves from the emotional burdens we carry. This freedom allows us to heal and reconcile not just with others but with ourselves. The act of forgiveness begins within, in the quiet space where we can meet our pain, acknowledge it, and then gently release it.

The heartbeat teaches us that reconciliation does not depend on external circumstances or on the actions of others. It arises from our own willingness to accept and embrace the full range of our emotions, letting go of what no longer serves us, and finding peace within ourselves.

As we reflect on our lives, the question of legacy often arises: *What will I leave behind? How will I be remembered?* The concept of legacy is not only about tangible achievements, but also about the relationships we nurture and the connections we make. MHbT offers a pathway to explore these questions, not through abstract or intellectual reflections, but through embodied presence.

Every heartbeat serves as a reminder to consider what we are offering the world in this moment. What relationships require attention? What words need to be spoken? What small acts of kindness can create lasting impact? Legacy, in the context of MHbT, is not about crafting a perfect story or leaving a flawless narrative. It is about fostering meaningful moments of connection, no matter how small, that will continue to echo in the hearts of those we love.

For families engaged in MHbT, the act of listening to a loved one's heartbeat becomes a deeply meaningful ritual. In these moments, the heartbeat becomes more than just a sound—it becomes a symbol of continuity. Even as life passes, the rhythm of the heart continues, offering comfort, connection, and love that transcends time.

For caregivers, the practice of reflecting on legacy can also prompt important questions about self-care. By focusing on the well-being of others, it is easy to overlook one's own needs. Yet the heartbeat reminds us that self-compassion and self-care are essential. They are not selfish, but necessary for sustaining the energy and love that caregivers offer to those they support. By caring for ourselves, we ensure that our presence remains a gift to others.

In a world that often prioritizes intellectual understanding and logical solutions, MHbT invites us to connect with a deeper form of wisdom—the wisdom of the body. The heart offers guidance that cannot be grasped through thinking alone but must be felt, experienced, and listened to.

Many who engage in MHbT speak of moments of clarity that arise not from intellectual reasoning but from the quiet presence of the body. By tuning into the heartbeat, individuals begin to trust their own inner guidance. The heart knows things that the mind does not, and through this practice, we learn to trust it. This embodied wisdom becomes a tool for decision-making, for healing, and for finding peace in moments of uncertainty.

For caregivers, this trust in the heart's wisdom offers a profound way to navigate the challenges of care. It teaches that simply being present—without needing to fix or solve—can be more powerful than any words or actions. In this presence, we offer comfort, connection, and understanding, not by providing answers, but by showing up fully, with open hearts.

MHbT is not only a personal journey; it is also a communal one. As patients, caregivers, and families come together to listen to the heartbeat, they create a shared rhythm—a rhythm that fosters connection, healing, and mutual understanding. In these communal spaces, the heartbeat becomes a bridge between individuals, reminding them that they are not alone.

The community cultivated through MHbT extends far beyond formal practice. It becomes a way of living—a practice of showing up for one another, of being present in the quiet moments of connection. Whether through shared silence, a touch, or a simple act of kindness, the rhythm of the heartbeat flows through all relationships. MHbT teaches us that healing is not an isolated experience—it is a collective one, nurtured by the presence and support of others.

As we reflect on the themes explored through the practice of MHbT, we are reminded that the heartbeat is more than just a physical sensation. It is a reminder of our connection to life itself—the ebb and flow, the beginning and end, the joy and sorrow. The heartbeat invites us to live fully in the present, embracing both the beauty and the challenges that come with being alive.

Take a moment now to place your hand over your heart. Feel the rhythm beneath your palm. With each beat, ask yourself: *What is this moment asking of me? What can I release? What can I embrace?* Know that as you listen to the heartbeat, you are part of a larger rhythm—one that connects you to yourself, to others, and to the great mystery of life.

As you continue through this journey, let each heartbeat be a reminder: *You are here. You are alive. And that is enough.* Let the rhythm of your heart carry you forward, through every challenge, every joy, and every moment of uncertainty. In that rhythm, may you find peace, presence, and the wisdom to live with open-hearted grace.

CHAPTER 8

CULTURAL DIVERSITY IN SPIRITUAL INTEGRATION AND MHBT

T he final heartbeat marks the end of a life, but across cultures the process of dying is much more than a biological event. It is a profound spiritual transition, rich with ritual and meaning. In every corner of the world, communities have developed ways to interpret and accompany the journey from life to death, often drawing on symbols and practices centered on the *heart* and its rhythms.

From the earliest times, humans recognized the heartbeat as the signature of life—the first drumbeat we hear in the womb, and the pulse that ceases at death. The heart has long been viewed as more than an organ; it is a universal symbol of vitality, emotion, and spirit. Ancient Egyptians, for instance, believed that the heart would be weighed in the afterlife to determine a soul's fate, literally balancing one's heart against the feather of truth to judge its purity. Many traditions similarly hold that the heart (or its beat) connects the material body with the immaterial soul: a liminal force at the threshold of life and death.

Equally universal is the use of *rhythm and sound* in end-of-life rites. Anthropologists emphasize that death is "a social event rather than the mere cessation of bodily functions," meaning that as the body's functions ebb, communities respond with ceremony—chants, prayers, drumming, songs—to honor the dying and guide their passage. The slow tolling of a bell at a Christian funeral, the steady drumbeat in an indigenous funeral dance, the chanting of Buddhist monks, or the recitation of a final prayer like the Jewish *Vidui* all use patterned sound or breath to sanctify the moment of death. In many cultures, such sounds are likened to heartbeats—uniting the gathered community's hearts in a common rhythm of mourning and hope.

This chapter explores cultural diversity in spiritual integration at the end of life, with a special focus on how different traditions engage the symbolism of the heart and the use of rhythm (heartbeat, music, breath) in dying rituals. We will journey through the wisdom of *Native American peoples* (especially New England tribes like the Pequot, Mohegan, and Algonquin), the rich teachings of *Buddhism* (Theravāda, Mahāyāna, and Tibetan Vajrayāna), the practices of *Christianity* (Catholic, Protestant, and contemplative mystical traditions), the customs of *Judaism* (Orthodox, Conservative, Reform, and Kabbalistic), and the perspectives of *global Indigenous communities* (from Andean highlands to Māori of Aotearoa to African traditional religions). For each, we examine how the process of dying is understood and ritualized: What is the role of the heart (literally and metaphorically)? How do rhythms—be it drumming, chanting, or breathing—facilitate the transition? What cosmologies of death and afterlife inform these practices? And how can a modern therapeutic approach like Meditative Heartbeat Therapy (MHbT) draw respectfully on these diverse traditions to support the spiritual well-being of the dying?

By comparing these traditions, we will uncover both striking commonalities and illuminating contrasts. Many share the recognition that in the final moments of life, something beyond the physical is at play—whether conceptualized as the soul, consciousness, or ancestral spirit. Many also use the language of the heart and the medium of rhythm to express compassion, continuity, and connection at the threshold of death. At the same time, each culture has unique rituals and beliefs: from the fire-lit vigils of New England's First Peoples to the elaborate chanting of Tibetan lamas, from the silent prayers of a Quaker vigil to the lively drum-dances of an Ashanti funeral.

The tone of this chapter is academic yet accessible. We draw on scholarly research, sacred texts, and oral histories to ground our exploration. Along the way, brief excerpts of prayers, chants, or legends give voice to how different peoples make meaning of death. While we do not present specific clinical case studies here, the insights gained are intended to guide practitioners of MHbT and others in integrating meditative heartbeat techniques with spiritual sensitivity at end-of-life. Ultimately, by learning how diverse cultures "ritualize and engage the process of dying" through the heart, we can deepen our own approach to accompanying the dying with respect, empathy, and a rhythm that resonates with the human spirit.

NATIVE AMERICAN TRADITIONS: THE HEARTBEAT OF THE EARTH AT LIFE'S END

Native American cultures are far from monolithic, yet many share a holistic view of life and death as interconnected parts of a sacred cycle. Death is often seen not as an end, but as a transition in which the spirit "walks on" into the next world. In some tribes, especially in the Southwest (e.g. Navajo and Apache), traditional beliefs cast death in a fearful light—the ghost of the dead might resent the living, so they performed swift, minimal ceremonies to send the spirit off and avoid lingering ghosts. By contrast, many other tribes—including those of the Northeast Woodlands like the Pequot, Mohegan, Algonquin, and Abenaki—view the spirits of the deceased as benevolent presences. Among these peoples, the dead are regarded as ever-present *ancestral spirits* who remain near their descendants. Dying is approached with acceptance or even a sense of continuity rather than dread.

For the Algonquian-speaking nations of New England, the heart and life-spirit are intimately linked to nature and the community.

Traditional cosmologies often held that each person's life was part of an ongoing fire or "flame" passed down from the ancestors. The individual's heart was seen as carrying this ancestral flame. When someone dies, it was common to keep a vigil fire burning by the body —not to destroy the remains, but to light the soul's way forward and to invite the ancestors to accompany the journey. The body (sometimes called the "shell" of the soul) would typically be buried in Mother Earth, often in a *flexed, fetal-like posture* and oriented eastward toward the rising sun, symbolizing eventual rebirth. Indeed, 17th-century accounts describe New England Algonquians wrapping the corpse in skins "with the knees against the stomach and the head on the knees, as we are in our mother's womb," then placing it in a deep grave in a seated fetal position. This burial posture was a sign of reverence and a return to the earth's womb. Mourners would sometimes place meaningful objects—weapons, tools, jewelry, even the deceased's dog—into the grave as *offerings and provisions* for the soul's journey, reflecting a belief that life continues in the spirit world much as in this one.

Far from fearing the departed, Northeastern tribes traditionally *honored* them. Family members and friends would demonstrate their grief openly. It was customary for relatives to paint their faces with black ash or charcoal as a visible mark of mourning— black being a sign of bereavement. Wakes or mourning ceremonies could last for days. In historical accounts, a dying person might be attended by loved ones who feasted in his presence, sang laments, and even gave him gifts to comfort him on his journey. Upon death, loud wails and "horrible cries" might be raised by the community—not only as expressions of grief but as calls reaching out to the spirit world. Among the Pequot and Mohegan, oral tradition holds that the departed remain near as guiding spirits; elders would speak of recently passed kin in the present tense, sensing their ongoing presence around the fires. The boundary between living and dead was permeable—"a veil thinner than a sheet of smoke"– and the heart-spirit of the person was expected to continue on in another form.

A poignant Mohegan story illustrates this view of death as transformation rather than destruction. In this tale, a warrior is killed in battle, leaving his young wife overcome with sorrow. Each night through the winter, she keeps a small fire burning beside his grave, tending it as carefully as one would a living heart. When spring arrives, a *red flower blooms* on that spot. To the Mohegan people, this was a sign that the warrior's love—the spiritual fire in his heart—had been reborn from the earth. Such stories convey the belief that the essence of a person (often symbolized by the heart or a flame) never truly dies; it returns to nature, to the community, and to the cycle of life in new ways.

The end-of-life rituals of Northeastern tribes reflected their beliefs in the ongoing life of the spirit and the need to send off the deceased with honor and guidance. Typically, before burial, a funeral ceremony would be held in the wigwam or lodge of the deceased. Elders or spiritual leaders (sometimes called an *autmoin* or medicine person) might lead prayers or dirges known as a "dead song" in the local language. These songs were often petitions addressed to the soul of the departed, guiding it on its journey. One observer noted that a chief would sing a *"death song"* as a prayer to the soul of the departed, first shortly after death and again at the grave when the body was interred. The assembled family and friends would join in these chants, accompanied by solemn drumming or rattle-shaking.

Music—especially *drumming*—held deep spiritual significance. In many Native American traditions, the drum's rhythm represents the heartbeat of the earth and the Creator. As Lucy Cannon-Neel (a Vermont Abenaki elder) explains, *"the drum is the heartbeat of Mother Earth"* and its pulse *"keeps everything... sound."* During communal rituals, whether in mourning ceremonies or seasonal gatherings, the steady beat of the drum was believed to align human hearts with the *great heart of the world*. Among Algonquin peoples, it is said that when people gathered around the funeral fire and the drum was played, "each individual heartbeat in the circle synchronizes with the drum's rhythm—many hearts beating as one. The drum, often called 'the heartbeat of Mother Earth,' thumps steadily, and everyone feels it in their chest." In such moments, the Earth's own heartbeat was felt to pulse through the drum, uniting the community with the ancestors in a single, living circle of connection. The drum's sound, along with chants and sacred dances, served as a bridge between the physical and spiritual realms. It was both an expression of grief and a way to strengthen the spiritual energy needed to send the departed peacefully onward.

Other ritual elements also emphasized *breath, rhythm, and guidance of the spirit*. For instance, some Northeastern tribes would light tobacco or sacred herbs, and the rising smoke (often fanned toward the east) was interpreted as carrying prayers heavenward and helping the soul ascend. In certain communities, a "death wail" or keening cry would be maintained in a rhythmic fashion by designated mourners for hours after the passing—almost like a musical chant of grief. The cadence of these wails could resemble breathing—a communal breathing out of sorrow.

Importantly, the community took great care of the body as the vessel that had carried the spirit. The deceased was dressed in their finest clothing and *wrapped carefully* (in bark or skins). They were not left alone; typically a vigil would be kept until burial, often with a fire or torch burning through the night as a sign of respect and guidance. This practice resonates with the contemporary concept of a hospice vigil or the Jewish *shmira* (watching the body)—an ancient acknowledgment that the end of life is a sacred time requiring presence and care.

In summary, Native American traditions such as those of the Pequot, Mohegan, and Algonquin illustrate a profound integration of the spiritual and natural dimensions of dying. The *heart*—both the literal organ and the metaphorical center of one's being—is central in their understanding of life's ebbing. It is tended with fire and song as a beloved flame that is passed on rather than extinguished. Through rhythmic drumming, chants, and reverent ceremony, these communities create a spiritual container for death that honors the individual, strengthens communal bonds, and reaffirms their connection to the Earth and ancestors.

For practitioners of Meditative Heartbeat Therapy, there is much to learn here. By recognizing the "heartbeat of Mother Earth" in the therapy space, one can create a culturally sensitive environment that respects indigenous patients' worldviews—for example, using soft drumming or recorded nature sounds during meditation, or simply acknowledging the presence of ancestors and the sacredness of the moment. The Native American approach teaches us that to help someone die well is not only to ease physical pain, but also to engage the rhythms of nature, the comfort of community, and the enduring heartbeat of spirit that continues beyond the final breath.

BUDDHIST TRADITIONS: HEART-MIND AND THE ART OF DYING

Buddhism approaches death with a clear-eyed recognition of *impermanence* (*anicca*) and an emphasis on the state of mind at the moment of death. Across Theravāda, Mahāyāna, and Vajrayāna (Tibetan) traditions, one finds diverse rituals—from serene mindfulness practices to elaborate chants—all aimed at ensuring a peaceful transition for the dying person's consciousness (*citta*). While Buddhism does not speak of a permanent soul or heart-spirit in the way some other religions do, it frequently uses the metaphor of the "heart" to mean the core of one's being (often equated with mind or awareness). Indeed, classical Theravāda theory locates the seat of consciousness in the region of the physical heart, known as the *hadaya-vatthu* or "heart-base." In this view, the heartbeat and the mind are subtly linked: the heart is the last support of consciousness in the dying process, and the rhythms of breath and pulse are integrated with mental states as one approaches the final breath.

In Theravāda Buddhist countries (such as Sri Lanka, Thailand, Myanmar, and Cambodia), end-of-life care often involves monks and family members jointly cultivating a calm and wholesome atmosphere for the dying person. There is a keen awareness that the *last conscious moments* can strongly influence the nature of one's rebirth. Thus, efforts are made to help the dying maintain a lucid, peaceful, and virtuous state of mind. Monks might lead the patient in reciting the *Three Refuges* (affirming faith in the Buddha, Dharma, and Sangha) or guide them in contemplating the Buddha's qualities. It is common for monks or relatives to chant verses from the Pāli scriptures. For example, the *Metta Sutta* (Buddha's discourse on loving-kindness) is frequently recited at deathbeds or funerals, radiating blessings of peace and goodwill to the departing person. The language of this chant directly speaks to the heart, encouraging the dying individual to let go of fear and to cultivate *mettā* (loving-kindness) for themselves and others, thus "opening the heart" at the moment of death.

Theravāda Buddhism also has specific contemplative practices for the dying. One such practice is *maranānussati* (mindfulness of death), wherein the person reflects on the naturalness of dying and the impermanence of the body. Skilled meditators sometimes focus on the sensation of the heartbeat or breath, observing it with equanimity until it fades. The heartbeat here serves as a final object of mindful attention—a kind of metronome counting down the last moments, to be watched without clinging. If fear or agitation arises, monks may remind the person to bring their awareness to the heart region and to cultivate *loving-kindness*, thus providing a gentle, heart-centered focus as physical life wanes.

Ritualistically, Theravāda communities often engage in *chanting and merit transfer* after a death. In countries like Thailand, it is customary for monks to chant passages from the *Abhidhamma* (the scholastic teachings) during the wake or funeral, which is believed to impart merit to the deceased and remind the living of the Buddha's wisdom. The chanting usually has a steady, sonorous cadence that creates a tranquil atmosphere. This "serene, meditative atmosphere" is believed to *calm the spirit of the deceased and aid in their journey*. In line with the doctrine of kamma (karma), the positive karma generated by chanting, offerings, and good thoughts is *dedicated* to the dying person to support a favorable rebirth.

In Theravāda understanding, at the very final moment of life, the mind consciousness (whose physical base is the heart) arises and ceases one last time, conditioning the first moment of consciousness in the next life. Therefore, if that last heartbeat is accompanied by mindfulness and compassion, it is considered extremely beneficial. There is a poignant scene often observed in Theravāda cultures: as a person is about to pass, those around may softly repeat phrases like "Buddho, Buddho" (evoking the Buddha) or chant the Refuges or verses of comfort. The dying, if conscious, might gently move their lips or simply listen. It is said in Buddhist tradition that *hearing is the last sense to fade*, so even if the person appears comatose, the rhythmic drone of Pāli chants or the familiar timbre of a teacher's voice can register in the heart-mind. In some Theravāda texts, there are instructions for attendants to literally speak into the dying person's left ear, reminding them of wholesome teachings and to focus on the Buddha. All these practices center on directing the "heart-mind" toward peace as the heartbeat slows and stops.

Mahāyāna Buddhist traditions in China, Japan, Korea, and Vietnam place great emphasis on collective ritual and the invocation of Buddhas and bodhisattvas at the time of death. Perhaps the most widespread practice is that of *Pure Land Buddhism*, wherein devotees aspire to be reborn in the Western Paradise of Amitābha (Amida) Buddha. In Pure Land belief, Amitābha has vowed that anyone who sincerely calls his name at the moment of death will be welcomed into his Pure Land. Therefore, at a dying person's bedside, it is common for family and monks to join in reciting *Namo Amitābhāya* (Homage to Amitābha Buddha) or simply Amitābha's name repeatedly. In Chinese, this is "*Namo Amituofo*," which devotees may chant hundreds of times in a soft, melodic repetition. This practice is known as *niànfó* (Buddha-recitation). As one scholar describes, it "creates a soundscape specific to the Pure Land deathbed," an environment where the name of Amitābha is ever-present. The dying person is urged to focus on Amitābha in their final moments; just hearing or calling out the Buddha's name with devotion is considered enough to ensure salvation in the Pure Land. Often those at the bedside will chant in unison, sometimes using rhythmic wooden fish drums or bells to maintain a steady beat. The collective rhythm serves both to keep the dying person's attention anchored and to generate a power-ful, heartfelt plea to Amitābha.

Traditional Pure Land scriptures vividly promise that Amitābha Buddha will appear at the deathbed of a faithful practitioner, some-times accompanied by saintly bodhisattvas, to guide their soul into the light. Thus, reports that a dying person sees a bright light or a vision of Buddha are taken as joyful confirmation that they will "have a good rebirth." These deathbed narratives reinforce the importance of chanting and faith. In practice, East Asian families today often play recordings of Amitābha's name or continue chanting around the clock for hours after a loved one has died, in case the consciousness is still in transition. In some Chinese communities, a group of lay chant-leaders (sometimes called *Buddhist friends*) can be invited to the home or hospital; they will chant *Amituofo* in shifts, creating an audi-tory cushion of compassion to carry the departing soul. The atmosphere is one of reverence and gentle optimism—tears are tempered by the belief that the deceased is going to a land of bliss. As one modern commentator notes, *"the act of chanting creates a serene, meditative atmosphere, which is believed to calm the spirit of the deceased and aid in their journey toward enlightenment,"* especially when the chant invokes Amitābha's blessings.

Apart from Pure Land practices, Mahāyāna traditions also use other chants and sutras to assist the dying and console the living. One of the most ubiquitous is the *Heart Sutra* (*Prajñā-pāramitā Hṛdaya Sūtra*), a short scripture on the emptiness of all phenomena. The Heart Sutra—ironically named, perhaps, since its teaching is that there is "no eye, no ear, no heart, no mind" that is permanent—is often recited at funerals in East Asia. In Japanese Zen monasteries, for example, monks will chant the Heart Sutra in Sino-Japanese, its rapid, rhythmic syllables filling the room. This sutra's famous lines, *"Form is emptiness, emptiness is form,"* remind all present that the phys-ical body is transient. Emptiness (*śūnyatā*) in Buddhism does not mean nihilism, but rather the interdependence and impermanence of all things. By chanting the Heart Sutra, mourners ritually acknowledge that the person who died has simply undergone a change of form.

As a Singapore Buddhist funeral guide explains, this chant *"emphasizes the impermanence of life* and helps the mourners come to terms with the transient nature of existence." It is believed that, on a spiritual level, the deceased may also benefit from hearing the truth of emptiness, helping them relinquish clinging to the last life and thus move onward without attachment.

Another common Mahāyāna practice is the chanting of the names of bodhisattvas known for their compassion. For instance, many Mahāyāna Buddhists chant the name of *Guanyin* (Avalokiteś-vara Bodhisattva) in times of fear and pain, including at the moment of death. The chant *"Namo Guanshiyin Pusa"* invokes the bodhisattva of Compassion to alleviate suffering and guide the soul safely. This is often accompanied by the use of prayer beads, keeping a steady count that can mirror the ticking of a clock or heartbeat—again using rhythm to focus the mind.

In summary, Mahāyāna Buddhism's end-of-life rites richly incorporate the symbolism of the heart and the power of rhythm. Whether it is the heartfelt calling of Amitābha's name or the steady cadence of a sutra, the goal is to engender the optimal mental state: calm, full of faith, and free of attachment. The "heart-mind" (*xin* in Chinese, which means both heart and mind) is nurtured through these practices to let go of this life gracefully and aspire to a higher spiritual plane. For a practitioner of MHbT, these Mahāyāna practices underscore the importance of sound and intention. One might, for example, integrate gentle mantra chanting or listen to recorded Buddhist chants during a heartbeat meditation for a Buddhist patient, aligning the therapeutic session with the client's spiritual frame of reference. Even the simple acknowledgement—"Let each heartbeat remind you of *Namo Amituofo*, of infinite light and compassion"—could resonate deeply for a Pure Land Buddhist facing death.

Tibetan Buddhism (Vajrayāna), with its elaborate teachings on death and rebirth, offers some of the most detailed spiritual maps for the end of life. In this tradition, death is a complex process involving the dissolution of the elements and consciousness into subtler states. Tibetan lamas often emphasize that *consciousness withdraws to the heart center at the time of death*. Esoteric teachings describe how the "white drop" from the crown and the "red drop" from the navel meet in the heart chakra at the moment of death, triggering the experience of the *Clear Light*—the fundamental luminosity of mind. This is considered a critical opportunity for liberation if recognized. In practical terms, Tibetan Buddhists consider the area of the heart to be especially sacred during and shortly after death, as it is the last locus of consciousness. A traditional Tibetan saying is that after the breath stops, "the consciousness dwells in the heart" for a time before leaving the body. For this reason, the body of a deceased monk or yogi is often left untouched (and not moved or disturbed) for three days, to allow the consciousness to depart peacefully. It is believed that rough handling—or even excessive displays of grief—too soon after death could startle the consciousness while it still lingers at the heart, potentially causing confusion for the departing soul.

The famous *Bardo Thodol*, popularly known as the *Tibetan Book of the Dead*, is essentially a guidebook for the consciousness of the deceased. Traditionally, a lama or knowledgeable person will read the *Bardo Thodol* text aloud near the corpse or dying person, to teach and remind the departing consciousness of the illusions it will face and how to move beyond fear. The text is rhythmic and chant-like. It literally addresses the dead person by name: *"O Nobly Born, now you are experiencing the Radiant Light of the Clear Mind of Death; recognize it..."* and so on. The belief is that, even if the person's gross ears have ceased to function, the subtle consciousness *hears these instructions*. This aligns with the idea (also present in Theravāda) that hearing is the last sense to fade; Tibetan tradition explicitly takes advantage of that by reciting guidance into the ear of the dying. A Buddhist teacher or family member might sit by the person's head and gently speak reminders: to let go of attachments, to trust in the compassionate Buddhas, and to move toward the Clear Light. This practice can be seen as a form of spiritual *entrainment*, not unlike MHbT's use of heartbeat sounds to entrain the mind into calm—here, the voice's steady cadence aims to entrain the departing mind into a state of clarity and fearlessness.

Another distinctive Tibetan practice is *Phowa* (transference of consciousness). In Phowa, a lama or trained practitioner performs a meditation at the moment of death (or soon after) to consciously "eject" the consciousness through the crown of the head, directing it toward a favorable rebirth (often Amitābha's Pure Land). The dying person may be coached to visualize their mind as a small orb of light moving from their heart upward and out the top of the head, riding on the syllable "HIK!" or propelled by mantra. If a lama is performing Phowa for someone else, they will often utter a sharp command or mantra, and sometimes a physical sign appears—a drop of blood or fluid at the crown—indicating success. Phowa is considered a highly advanced practice, but in Tibet it became part of folk custom too: local villagers might call a lama to do Phowa for a relative who had just died. The key here is the idea that the *heart consciousness can be propelled by ritual rhythm* (a focused mantra or chant) and by compassionate intent into a higher state. It is another example of how rhythm (in this case the rhythm of a mantra and visualization) is used at the threshold of death.

During Tibetan funerals and cremation ceremonies, we also see rich rhythmic and musical elements. Monks use *dungchen* (long trumpets), *cymbals*, and *damaru* (hand drums) to create a powerful sonic environment. The deep drone of the dungchen and the staccato crack of drums are not merely music; they are considered offerings to buddhas and wrathful deities, and simultaneously they "shake loose" any clinging the soul might have to the earthly realm, driving it forward. The heartbeat-like thump of the damaru, often accompanied by the eerie wail of the kangling (a trumpet made from a human thigh bone), confronts the reality of impermanence in a visceral way. For the Tibetan mind, these sounds are reminders that the body is but a vessel—now empty—and the consciousness must journey on.

Central to Tibetan Buddhism's approach is the concept of the *bardo*, the intermediate state between death and rebirth, traditionally said to last up to 49 days. As noted in a Singapore Mahāyāna context, "the soul remains in a transitional state, known as bardo... for up to 49 days after death." Tibetans take this interim seriously and perform weekly prayers (every 7 days) until the 49th day, dedicating merit to the departed. They may sponsor the printing of holy texts, the lighting of butter lamps (analogous to keeping a flame of consciousness), and the recitation of the deceased's favorite prayers or mantras. The *rhythm of these ceremonies*—held on specific days—is thought to help the wandering consciousness gradually find its way. Each ritual is like a heartbeat in the post-mortem interim, a regular pulse of compassion sent to the one who has passed on.

From a modern therapeutic perspective, Tibetan Buddhism offers a profoundly detailed model of how to assist someone in the dying process. It underscores the importance of maintaining a *peaceful, controlled environment* where the dying person's inner experience is carefully guided. The use of the voice, of mantra, of breathing techniques (Tibetan yogis sometimes train to take a final conscious breath and then enter a deep meditation as they die), all resonate with the principles of MHbT. For example, a practitioner of MHbT working with a Tibetan Buddhist client might incorporate visualization techniques drawn from Phowa—perhaps inviting the person, during a heartbeat meditation, to imagine each heartbeat as a step closer to the light at the top of their head, preparing for a graceful exit. Or they might simply ensure that after the client's death, caregivers know of the Tibetan custom to allow the body to rest untouched for a period, or to play soft chants (such as *Om Mani Padme Hum*) in the room, respecting the belief that the "inner ear" of the heart may still be listening.

In conclusion, Buddhism provides a rich array of end-of-life practices that revolve around training the mind (or heart-mind) at the crucial juncture of death. Whether through mindfulness and loving-kindness in Theravāda, devotional chanting in Mahāyāna, or intricate tantric rites in Vajrayāna, the themes of heartbeat and rhythm are subtly present—as metaphors, as tools, and as natural phenomena to be heeded. All these practices share the goal of easing the transition out of this life with awareness and compassion. The heartbeat meditation of MHbT, when adapted with cultural sensitivity, can complement these practices by offering a *universal bridge*: helping Buddhist patients of any tradition find focus and comfort in the familiar rhythm of life as they prepare for its gentle cessation.

CHRISTIAN PERSPECTIVES:
THE HEART'S FAITH AND THE RITUALS OF FAREWELL

In Catholic Christianity, the end of life is accompanied by rich sacramental rituals designed to offer grace, forgiveness, and solace to the dying. The *"Last Rites"* (more formally, Viaticum and the Anointing of the Sick, often preceded by Confession) are a final ministry of the Church to its member. A priest anoints the person's forehead and hands with holy oil, laying hands on them and praying for the Holy Spirit's healing and forgiveness. The very term *Viaticum* means "provision for the journey," referring to the last Communion received by the dying as spiritual food for the passage through death. The purpose of these rites is to *prepare the soul for death and to give peace to the mind*. There is a profound trust that through these sacraments, Christ himself fortifies the person's heart: sins are absolved, fears are calmed, and the person is united with Jesus' suffering and resurrection.

During the administration of last rites, prayers specifically invoke the heart and mercy of Jesus. For example, a short traditional aspiration often prayed at a Catholic deathbed is: *"Heart of Jesus, once in agony, have mercy on the dying."* This simple invocation captures a core Christian belief: that Jesus, whose Sacred Heart burns with love, accompanies the dying person in their agony and opens for them the door to eternal life. The image of the *Sacred Heart of Jesus*—a heart encircled by thorns, yet radiating light—is a powerful Catholic symbol of Christ's compassionate presence, especially in suffering and death. Many devout Catholics, in their final moments, clutch a crucifix or a Sacred Heart medal, feeling the nearness of Jesus' love. Similarly, prayers to the Virgin Mary, such as the *Ave Maria*, ask for her intercession "now and at the hour of our death," highlighting an emotional reliance on maternal comfort at life's end.

The Eastern Orthodox Church shares many of the same sacraments (often called "Mysteries") for the dying: it offers Holy Unction (anointing) and final Holy Communion. Orthodox last prayers include the *Canon for the Departure of the Soul*, in which the priest and family commend the person to God. In these prayers, the imagery of light and heart is also present—asking Christ to receive the soul into His hands and to place it in *"Abraham's bosom"* (a term for heavenly rest). Orthodox Christian funerary tradition is richly musical: the haunting hymn *"Memory Eternal"* (*Vichnaya Pamyat*) is sung, its deep, slow intonations almost mimicking the steady toll of a bell or a heartbeat. This repeated chant expresses the hope that God will remember the departed in His heart forever, and it has a hypnotic, consoling effect on mourners who may join in the refrain.

Another Orthodox hymn, *"Give rest, O Lord, to the soul of Thy servant,"* is set to a solemn, repetitive melody that can induce a meditative state. The use of these chants demonstrates the Christian understanding that through sacred sound and ritual, the community can lift the soul heavenward. The *rhythm of prayer*—whether the litanies intoned by a priest or the call-and-response of the rosary—provides spiritual structure at a time when the dying person and their loved ones might otherwise feel chaos or despair.

One cannot speak of Christian end-of-life spirituality without mentioning the image of the *Cross*. In Catholic and Orthodox rooms, the dying often gaze upon a crucifix. Many will literally hold a crucifix over their heart as they pass. In doing so, they unite their own final heartbeats with the heartbeat of Jesus on the cross—whose human heart, Christians believe, stopped on Good Friday only to beat again in glory on Easter. The symbolism of Jesus' heart—pierced and then resurrected—offers believers hope that death is not the final word. Thus, in Catholic and Orthodox rituals, the heart is omnipresent: in theological language (the Sacred Heart, the Immaculate Heart of Mary), in emotional tenor (heartfelt prayers, acts of contrition from the heart), and even in physicality (holy water is sprinkled, making the sign of the cross over the heart of the dying). All these serve to comfort and encourage the dying person to "give their heart to God" in trust.

It's worth noting that the very word *"courage"* comes from the Latin *cor* (heart). At the Christian deathbed, clergy often pray for God to give the dying person "courage and peace." In the Commendation of the Dying (a set of prayers said at the moment of death), the priest prays: *"Go forth, O Christian soul, in the name of God the Father Almighty who created you, in the name of Jesus Christ, Son of the living God, who suffered for you, in the name of the Holy Spirit who was poured out upon you. ... May you live in peace this day, may your home be with God in Zion."* The repetitive invocation of the Trinity and blessings functions almost like a mantra of release. Many times, those around the bed will join by softly saying *"Amen"* or *"Jesus, mercy"* in rhythm with the priest's prayers. The dying person's breaths may become labored, but the prayer rhythm provides a kind of entrainment—a steady, hopeful pattern to cling to, much like a lullaby as one "falls asleep" in death.

From a medical perspective, these Catholic and Orthodox practices often have observable calming effects. The familiar cadence of the rosary or the anointing prayers can lower anxiety for the dying and family alike. Studies in pastoral care note that patients often visibly relax when the rites of their faith are performed—tears that flow are often tears of release, not distress. In essence, the Church's rituals speak to the *heart*: they reaffirm the person's dignity and belovedness in the eyes of God, helping to dispel the loneliness and fear that can plague the end of life.

Protestant Christianity encompasses a wide range of denominations and practices, but several common themes emerge in end-of-life care: reliance on *Scripture reading*, the offering of *extemporaneous prayer*, the singing of favorite *hymns*, and an emphasis on personal trust in God's promises. Unlike Catholic and Orthodox Christians, most Protestants do not have a fixed set of "last rites" or required clerical rituals (with the partial exception of some Anglicans and Lutherans who retain a form of anointing or commendation).

Instead, the moments around death are often marked by simplicity and deep personalism.

It is typical in Protestant families that as a loved one is dying, someone might read from the Bible at the bedside. Classic choices include *Psalm 23* ("The Lord is my shepherd... Even though I walk through the valley of the shadow of death, I will fear no evil...") and passages from the Gospels such as *John 14:1–3*, where Jesus says, *"Let not your hearts be troubled... In my Father's house are many mansions... I will come again and will take you to myself."* Such verses explicitly address the heart—"let not your heart be troubled"—offering comfort and hope. The rhythm of biblical language, especially in traditional translations like the King James Bible, has a solemn, steadying cadence that many find soothing. Family or clergy might also recite the *Lord's Prayer* together, its measured meter ("Our Father, who art in heaven...") creating a unity of voices and hearts.

One of the great treasures of Protestant heritage is its *hymnody*. Hymns are frequently sung or played in the dying hours. Many hospice nurses can recount instances of a family softly singing *"Amazing Grace"* or *"Nearer, My God, to Thee"* as a patient took their last breaths. These hymns often have a slow, heartbeat-like tempo and comforting lyrics. For example, "Amazing Grace," in its final verse, affirms: *"When flesh and heart shall fail, and mortal life shall cease, I shall possess within the veil, a life of joy and peace."* In fact, a well-known line from a Protestant hymn, *"It Is Well with My Soul,"* was written by Horatio Spafford after great tragedy and is often sung at funerals: *"When peace like a river attendeth my way... It is well, it is well with my soul."* Singing these lines can bring a *palpable peace* to the room—the communal act of singing regulates breathing and can even synchronize heartbeats among those present (a phenomenon observed in choral settings). The dying person, if conscious, might hum along or simply relax into the melody. In cases where the dying person is unresponsive, families often report that their loved one seemed to pass away more tranquilly during or just after a beloved hymn was sung, almost as if the soul was carried upward on the notes.

Spontaneous prayer is another hallmark of Protestant end-of-life practice. Without a set liturgy, ministers or family members will pray from the heart in plain language. Common themes include thanking God for the person's life, affirming the hope of heaven through Jesus, and asking God to receive the person. For Evangelical Protestants, a key concern is the individual's personal relationship with Jesus. Thus, if a person is conscious and able, a pastor might gently lead them in reaffirming their faith—essentially, ensuring the person "*confesses with their mouth and believes in their heart*" (cf. Romans 10:9) one last time. There is the well-known Evangelical concept of "accepting Jesus into your heart." In the context of dying, this might be expressed as an earnest prayer: "*Lord Jesus, I (or he/she) entrust my heart to You now. Come and live in me forever.*" For those who are already devout, the language may focus on assurance: "*Lord, into Your hands we commend this dear brother's spirit.*" Protestants draw direct inspiration from Jesus' own last words on the cross: "*Father, into your hands I commend my spirit*" (Luke 23:46). This act of *entrustment* is essentially a heart-action—a final giving of one's heart and soul back to God who gave it.

The environment at a Protestant deathbed may be less formally ritualized than in Catholic settings, but it is often rich with personal touches. A common practice in some communities is the sharing of favorite *Bible verses or hymns* by those gathered, almost like a vigil. Each person might take a turn quoting a promise of God that is meaningful: "*He will never leave you nor forsake you,*" "*I go to prepare a place for you,*" "*Who shall separate us from the love of Christ?... neither death nor life... will be able to separate us from the love of God*" (Romans 8:38–39). These recitations act as verbal talismans against fear. They reinforce in the dying person's heart the core Protestant conviction of salvation by faith and God's unbreakable love.

In many Protestant funerals (which often occur days after death), the tone is set as a "celebration of life" and a confident committal of the person to God. But even before death, one can see this ethos: some individuals, aware that death is near, turn their dying days into a time of reconciliation, testimony, and even song. There are accounts of Methodists in the 18th–19th centuries gathering around a dying friend and singing Charles Wesley's hymns to "sing them into heaven." This tradition of *deathbed singing* continues in various forms; for example, members of certain Mennonite communities offer "choral hospice care" where small groups sing quiet a cappella hymns for the dying, bringing a sense of sacred calm.

For Protestants, the *heart's state of trust* is paramount. There is a strong belief that what saves a person is their heartfelt faith in Christ. Thus, the greatest concern is that the person dies "at peace with God," having trusted Jesus as Savior. Once that is assured (or presumed), the practices around are meant to console and encourage. The use of the heart metaphor is frequent in prayers: one might pray that God "comfort the hearts" of the family, or that the dying person's heart be filled with God's presence. Unlike some Eastern religions, there isn't usually an attempt to match breathing or heartbeat to specific prayers—however, many hospice caregivers observe that playing *soft Christian hymns* or worship music can lead to a more regular breathing pattern in agitated patients. In essence, the music and words provide an external rhythm that the person can subconsciously latch onto, slowing their physiological rhythms into a more peaceful state. This is quite analogous to how MHbT uses the heartbeat as an anchor—in Protestant spirituality, it is often the steady rhythm of a well-known Psalm or the lilting meter of *"The Lord is my shepherd"* that serves as the anchor for a dying person's consciousness.

In summary, Protestant end-of-life practices center on *Scripture (the Word)* and *Song*, delivered in a personal, heartfelt manner. They aim to saturate the dying person's mind and heart with reminders of God's love and the promise of eternal life. The role of community is also vital: the gathered family's shared prayers or singing create a field of spiritual support that can carry the individual on their final journey. This communal aspect resonates with the idea in MHbT that a supportive presence—and perhaps a gentle rhythmic cue like soft music or spoken prayer—can alleviate anxiety at the end of life. A culturally sensitive application of MHbT for a Protestant Christian might incorporate gentle hymn tunes played in the background as the person focuses on their heartbeat, or the facilitator might quietly recite a Psalm in time with the person's breathing, merging bodily rhythm with spiritual verse.

Beneath and beyond denominational differences, Christianity harbors an ancient stream of contemplative practice that directly engages the heart and its rhythms. In the Eastern Orthodox tradition, this is epitomized by *Hesychasm*, the practice of inner stillness and the continuous praying of the *Jesus Prayer*: *"Lord Jesus Christ, Son of God, have mercy on me."* Hesychast monks since at least the 4th century taught methods to synchronize this short prayer with one's *breath and heartbeat.* The goal was to internalize the prayer so deeply that it "descends from the mind into the heart," becoming as natural and constant as one's heartbeat. As one modern summary puts it, *"Some [Christian mystics] link this prayer to the breath, heartbeat, prostrations, or thoughts of death."* By aligning the prayer with the beating of the heart and the flow of breathing, the person enters a profound state of coherence—mentally, physically, and spiritually unified. This is strikingly parallel to certain meditative practices in Eastern religions and indeed to the principles of MHbT.

At the time of death, these contemplative practices offer powerful tools for spiritual integration. An Orthodox Christian who has practiced the Jesus Prayer through their life may naturally fall into its rhythm as they die. There are accounts of elderly monks passing away with the words *"Lord Jesus... mercy..."* softly moving on their lips until they stopped mid-phrase, as if seamlessly transitioning their prayer from this world to the next. The *Prayer of the Heart* (as the Jesus Prayer is often called) is believed to invoke the presence of Christ in the innermost self. Dying while immersed in this prayer is considered an ideal "falling asleep in the Lord." Even for those not formally trained in Hesychasm, the concept is accessible: chaplains sometimes encourage Christian patients to synchronize a short prayer or holy name with their breath as a form of anxiety relief. For example, breathing in with "Lord Jesus" and breathing out with "have mercy" can slow the heart rate and center the mind on the divine. Many hospice patients, even without knowing the term *Hesychasm*, find comfort in holding a cross or rosary and internally repeating a beloved prayer rhythmically—in effect, performing a personal form of the prayer of the heart.

Catholic contemplative saints also wrote about offering one's final sufferings as a *"prayer of the heart"* to God. St. Thérèse of Lisieux, for instance, on her deathbed in 1897, spoke of her heart being filled with love to offer to Jesus as she died; she famously said, *"I am not dying; I am entering life."* She had a custom of attuning her simple aspirations ("Jesus, I love you") to the rhythm of daily activities; at death, this translated into aligning her fading breaths with trust in God. Such examples illustrate that, across Christianity, there exists a thread of using the body's natural rhythms—heartbeat and breath—as a scaffold for prayerful attention, especially in confronting mortality.

Quaker Christians (the Society of Friends) provide another contemplative model. In Quaker tradition, communal worship often happens in *silence*, with the belief that God speaks directly to each heart in the stillness. At a Quaker's deathbed, it is not uncommon for family and Friends to sit in a silent vigil, creating a palpable field of prayer without words. In that silence, the only sounds might be the ticking of a clock or the faint breathing of the patient—essentially highlighting those basic rhythms. After a period of silence, individuals may feel moved to speak a gentle message or sing a verse of a hymn, but then they return to silence. This ebb and flow resembles a heartbeat in itself: sound and quiet in natural alternation. The Quaker approach underscores profound *listening*—listening with the "ear of the heart" for God's guidance. For a dying person, this can be very comforting, as it removes pressure to speak or do anything, and simply offers loving presence. It resonates with the MHbT emphasis on presence and mindfulness: being fully present to the heartbeat of the moment.

In Eastern Orthodox Christianity, there is also a practice of reading or chanting the *Psalms* continuously around the body from death until burial (often a 2-day vigil). This is contemplative in that the chant of the Psalms (especially Psalm 119, a favorite at Orthodox funerals) is done in a soft, monotone manner that is almost like a drone. Mourners sitting by the coffin may synchronize their quiet prayer (like the Jesus Prayer) to the drone of the psalmody. The effect is soothing and deeply spiritual; it creates an atmosphere that acknowledges death while bathing it in the poetry of faith. The repetition of phrases like "The Lord is compassionate and merciful" or "Into Your hands I commend my spirit" throughout the Psalms can imprint those truths onto the consciousness of all present.

From a practical standpoint, Christian contemplative traditions offer techniques that could be incorporated into meditative heartbeat therapy for those who share that faith background. For example, encouraging a patient to match a short prayer to their heartbeat (if that is comforting for them) can be a way of integrating their spirituality with the therapeutic process. One could invite a patient to gently place a hand on their heart and feel its beating, and perhaps say internally with each beat, *"Jesus... Jesus..."* or *"Peace... be with me."* This is not unlike a mantra meditation, but framed in the patient's own religious language. As noted in an Orthodox source, *"the mind should be in the heart,"* offering up prayer from the depths of the heart—an approach like this can facilitate exactly that: uniting thought, breath, and heartbeat in a single spiritual act.

IN CONCLUSION, Christianity—through its sacraments, scriptures, songs, and silent prayers—provides a rich tapestry of end-of-life practices centered on comforting the heart and entrusting it to God. The theme of the heart runs through it all: hearts contrite in repentance, hearts courageous in faith, hearts united with the divine heart of Jesus, hearts lifted by melody and soothed by prayer. The use of rhythm, whether through formal liturgy or spontaneous hymnody or the steady silent prayer of a mystic, is a means to synchronize the believer's soul with the eternal. For a therapy like MHbT that uses the literal heartbeat as a focus, the alignment with Christian spiritual rhythms can be very natural. A sensitive practitioner will find that by accommodating a patient's inclination to prayer or sacred music during sessions, the therapeutic and the spiritual will reinforce each other, leading the person to an integrated peace—truly making "a joyful noise" in the heart even in life's final movement.

JEWISH PERSPECTIVES ON DEATH AND THE HEART

In Jewish tradition, death is approached with reverence, community support, and a focus on the oneness of body and soul. Judaism places strong emphasis on the *heart* as the seat of understanding and devotion (the Hebrew word *lev* often means "heart/mind"), and this symbolism carries into end-of-life rituals. A dying person in Jewish practice is treated with utmost dignity, and the moments around death are filled with prayer and love. The Talmud teaches that one should not abandon a person who is *goses* (actively dying), highlighting the deep value of presence at the deathbed.

Traditional Prayers and Vigil: When death is imminent, it is customary for family and friends to gather and ensure the person is not alone. A central practice is the recitation of the *Vidui*, or deathbed confession. This prayer, said by the dying person or someone on their behalf, is a final act of repentance and affirmation of faith. A version of the Vidui reads: I acknowledge before You, my God and God of my ancestors, that my healing and my death are in Your hands... if I die, may my death be an atonement for all my sins before You, and may my portion be in Paradise and my soul bound up in the bond of life." The Vidui is uttered "with a dying breath," reconciling the soul with the Creator in a spirit of oneness. Often, those gathered will gently prompt the dying person to affirm the *Shema* ("Hear O Israel, the Lord is our God, the Lord is One"), the most fundamental declaration of faith. Saying *Shema Yisrael* with one's last breath is considered a great merit—many Jewish martyrs throughout history died with "Adonai Echad" ("the Lord is One") on their lips.

As the soul is believed to depart with the final breath, there are traditional verses and sayings to mark that exact moment. A beautiful custom is to recite biblical verses that release the soul: *"Go in peace, and may you rest on the wings of the Divine Presence." Another set of lines invokes the *angels* to accompany the person: *"May Michael be at your right, Gabriel at your left... and the Shekhinah (Divine Presence) above your head." These verses, often chanted in soft tones, create a *sacred rhythm* at the moment of passing—a litany of protection as the heart's earthly labor ends. It is notable that some of these verses explicitly mention the heart: *"Be strong and of good courage, do not fear... for your God is with you wherever you go." This is both a scriptural quote (Joshua 1:9) and a direct encouragement to the dying person's heart not to be afraid.

Care for Body and Soul: In Jewish thought, the soul (*neshamah*) is the God-given life-breath, and it returns to God at death, while the body (sometimes called the person's "garment" or vessel) must be treated with respect. Immediately after death, a practice called *Shmirah* (guarding) begins: friends or community members act as *shomrim* (guardians), staying with the body and often reciting Psalms continuously until burial. This practice recognizes that something sacred remains—it is said that a *ruach* (spirit or aura) lingers with the body until burial. Thus the communal heartbeat continues around the deceased; the reading of Psalms has its own gentle rhythm that fills the silence. Psalm 23 is commonly read, as are others like Psalm 91 and Psalm 121, whose verses (e.g., *"The Lord will guard your going and coming, now and forever"*) speak to trust in God's sheltering heart. This vigil is an act of love that soothes the grief of those present as much as it is believed to soothe the departing soul, creating an atmosphere where, as one Jewish text puts it, *"the soul is not bewildered by loneliness."*

Jews do not traditionally employ music or overt rhythmic elements in funeral rites; instead, *chanting of scripture* and *eulogies* (which often have their own cadences) set the tone. However, the absence of instrumental music can itself be seen as a kind of reverent rhythm—the natural sounds of tears, the tearing of kri'ah (garments) by mourners, the shoveling of earth on the grave—all form part of the soundscape of mourning. One notable heart-centered custom: after burial, those at the cemetery form two lines, and the mourners pass between them to receive comfort. As they do, the community often recites the words *"HaMakom yenachem etchem..."* meaning "May the Omnipresent One comfort you among the mourners of Zion and Jerusalem." The communal recitation of this phrase, again and again to each mourner, is like a heartbeat of compassion extended to the bereaved.

Mystical Perspectives: In Kabbalistic (mystical) Judaism, the heart and breath take on special significance at death. Kabbalah speaks of multiple levels of soul—*nefesh* (life force), *ruach* (spirit/wind), *neshamah* (higher soul)—that depart in stages. The *nefesh*, associated with blood and the body, remains with the corpse until burial; the *ruach* hovers for seven days near the home; the *neshamah* returns to its divine source. This gradation underscores why the body is treated as "still connected" to the person for some time. Some Kabbalistic texts describe death for the righteous as a "kiss of God," wherein the soul leaves through a kiss—symbolically through the mouth (breath) or perhaps the heart. Indeed, it is said that Moses, Aaron, and Miriam died by the *"kiss of the Shekhinah."* This poetic image conveys an effortless, gentle separation of soul and body, akin to a flame being extinguished with a soft breath. It frames death not as violence to life but as an intimate act of union with the Divine. In practical terms, Kabbalists strongly discourage excessive displays of grief that might disturb the soul's journey; instead, they encourage *focused prayer* and *tzedakah* (charity) in the deceased's merit, which are thought to elevate the soul and ease its passage.

The Jewish approach to end-of-life shows a deep concern for the *heart and soul's peace.* From the Vidui that clears the conscience, to the Shema affirming faith with one's whole heart, to the tender guarding of the body, every element is meant to comfort and guide. The Hebrew word for *compassion—rachamim—*is linked to *rechem* (womb). In death, the community in a sense creates a womb of compassion around the dying, encircling them with prayer and presence so they can be "born" into the next world. The heartbeat of that womb is the steady cadence of blessings, the quiet Psalm recitations, and the cultural rhythms of ritual (meal after the funeral, seven days of *shiva* mourning, thirty days of *sheloshim*, and so on—structured time that gives mourners a rhythm to follow).

For modern therapeutic contexts, Jewish practices highlight the importance of *verbal prayer and vigil*. A Jewish patient might draw comfort from simply having the Psalms playing softly (many enjoy sung or spoken Psalms) or the presence of a chaplain to say the Vidui if family cannot. If integrating MHbT, one might invite a patient to place a hand on their heart and silently recite a short prayer in Hebrew or their preferred language in sync with their heartbeat—much like some observant Jews feel the pulse when saying "El Na Refa Na La" (a biblical healing plea) on behalf of the sick, treating the pulse like a prayer drum. The key is to respect the *quiet sanctity* often preferred in Jewish dying moments (no flamboyant additions), and to use gentle reminders of God's mercy (for example, recalling *"Though my flesh and heart fail, God is the strength of my heart,"* from Psalm 73:2).

In essence, Judaism teaches that at death, the *heart and soul return to God* who gave them (echoing Ecclesiastes 12:7). The rituals are designed to make that return one of peace, forgiveness, and connection. The heart stops, but it stops in the hope of divine embrace. As the traditional epitaph says in Hebrew, *"Tehe nishmato tzrurah bitzror ha-chayim"*—"May his soul be bound up in the bond of life." This expresses the belief that the departed heart is not lost, but bound into the living heart of the community and the eternal life of God.

GLOBAL INDIGENOUS PERSPECTIVES: RHYTHMS OF CONTINUITY AND SACRED HEARTBEATS

Across diverse indigenous cultures of the world—from the mountains of the Andes to the islands of the Pacific and the villages of Africa—we find varied understandings of death, yet common threads emerge. These traditions often view death not as an extinction but as a *transition to the realm of ancestors or spirits*, and they employ communal rituals, music, and symbolism to honor this passage. The *heartbeat of drums*, the cadence of chants, and the controlled breath of song or dance play crucial roles in these final rites, serving to connect the living and the dead in a shared spiritual space.

In the high Andes, where indigenous Quechua and Aymara cosmologies persist (often syncretized with Catholicism), death is seen as a journey of the soul through a sacred landscape. Ethnohistoric accounts describe how, after death, the spirit (*aya*) must travel a difficult road to reach the land of the ancestors. One traditional Quechua belief holds that the soul comes to a deep canyon with a raging river known as the *"River of Blood" (Yawar Mayu)*. To cross safely, the spirit must enlist the help of a *black dog*—a mystical guide —who leads it over a bridge of human hair to the other side. Once across, the soul passes through different mystical villages and high plateaus, finally arriving at a *mountain deity* (an Apu) who guards the gateway to the ancestral real. Christian influence introduced images like *San Francisco* (St. Francis) waiting at the mountaintop gate, blending native and Catholic elements. These beliefs illustrate a view of death as a *path to be traversed*, requiring guidance and ritual assistance.

Andean funerary practices historically involved extensive ritual and rhythmic elements. In Inca and pre-Inca times, it was common to maintain relationships with the departed through the preservation of mummies and periodic ceremonies. Even today, rural Andean communities observe *Todos Santos* (All Saints/Day of the Dead) with unique traditions: families may play specific melancholic melodies on flutes or guitars to call spirits of ancestors to partake in ceremonial foods. During funerals, music is present as well. For example, among some Aymara communities, *panpipe ensembles* (known as *sikus*) play dirges during the wake, their low, breathy harmonies thought to *attract ancestral spirits* to accompany the soul. The pulsating sound of panpipes—which require circular breathing, creating a continuous wave of sound—can feel like a sonic metaphor for the continuity of life, a musical heartbeat connecting generations.

A fascinating aspect of some Andean beliefs is the idea that humans possess *multiple souls or soul-essences*. In certain Quechua communities, it's said a person has more than one soul: one (sometimes called *aya* or *shaya*) that leaves the body at death to journey onward, and another that stays with the bones or tomb (*corporeo* or *sombra*) as a protective presence. One Spanish chronicler noted that some Andean villagers claimed a man has three souls and a woman as many as seven—reflecting, perhaps, the high esteem for women's spiritual resilience (as they endure childbirth). At a death, the community would often make loud rhythmic sounds—beating on walls or loud keening—not only to announce the passing but to *help send off the departing soul* and to scare away any harmful spirits. Personal belongings were buried with the dead to help the soul in its journey, similar to ancient Egyptian or Chinese custom. To this day, Andean families will bury favorite items (hat, coca leaf pouch, tools) with their loved one, acknowledging that the person's *heart desires* should be cared for even in death.

Andean worldview integrates natural cycles—day/night, seasonal rhythms—with the journey of souls. An old Quechua saying holds that"When it is day for us, it is night for the souls; when it is night for us, it is day for them." Thus, many rituals for the dead happen at twilight or dawn, liminal times to help the soul in its own reversal of day and night. The *heart*, in Andean thought, is not anatomically singled out as the seat of the soul (indeed, the Quechua word *sonqo* means "heart" but implies the whole inner self). But metaphorically, there is a focus on *"keeping the fire of the heart alive."* For example, it was common (and still is in some communities) to maintain a *"funeral fire"* next to the body or coffin throughout the wake. This fire is often fed with wood and sustained through the night. Symbolically, it represents the *heart-flame* of the person and the ancestors. In fact, a practice among some Quechua is to take a *small coal* from this fire after the funeral and use it to start the hearth fire back at home—literally carrying the deceased's flame into the living space. This resonates strongly with the notion of continuity: the individual heart's fire joins the larger ancestral fire in the community hearth. *"Each of us carries the flames of our forebears in our heart, and we will pass that on to those after us,"* as one Andean perspective puts it.

For an outside observer, Andean death rites demonstrate how *earth, heart, and community* are bound together. The use of drums (some Andean communities use a large drum called *tinya* in funeral marches), flutes, and constant vigil lights shows an intuitive understanding that *rhythm and light guide the soul.* These practices certainly comfort the living too, giving them active roles—making music, tending fire—to channel grief.

In applying these insights, a therapist might find that Andean clients take comfort in *ritual action.* Integrating that into therapy could be as simple as lighting a small candle (an echo of the vigil fire) during sessions or encouraging the patient's family to perform any small ritual they find meaningful (like quietly singing an Andean lullaby or prayer while the patient focuses on their heartbeat). The imagery of the living and the dead separated by a veil thinner than a sheet of smoke" (as one Mohegan story put it) could be relatable to Andean clients too, given their use of fire and smoke as connecting elements. Thus, an Andean patient might be invited to imagine, with each heartbeat, a warm light glowing (like a fire coal) in their heart that connects to their loved ones—a visualization aligned with their cultural symbols.

For the Māori people of Aotearoa (New Zealand), death is not an endpoint but part of a *continuum* between the seen and unseen worlds. Māori believe that the spirit (*wairua*) continues after death and eventually makes a journey back to the ancestral homeland. According to Māori lore, when someone dies, their wairua travels to the westernmost tip of the North Island, to Te Rerenga Wairua (Cape Reinga)*. There, a revered pohutukawa tree clings to the cliff. It is said the spirits slide down a root of this tree into the sea, then journey onward to *Hawaiki,* the mythic homeland from which Māori ancestors came. Along the way, at a point called *Te Ārai ("the Veil"),* spirits pause and look back to *whenua* (the land, home) one last time, sometimes reluctant to depart. Only after this farewell do they leap off toward Hawaiki. This cosmology frames Māori end-of-life rituals: the process of dying is a *spiritual voyage*, and those left behind must send their loved one off properly and support their wairua's journey.

The Māori funeral rite, or *Tangihanga (Tangi)*, is among the most elaborate and community-centered in the world. It typically unfolds over three days on a *marae* (tribal meeting ground). The deceased's body (often adorned with fine woven cloaks and treasures) lies in state, and around it the people gather day and night. *Rituals of encounter* structure the Tangihanga: when visitors arrive to pay respects, women perform a *karanga* (a ceremonial call)—an eerie, rising chant that *weaves together a greeting to the living and a call to the spirit of the deceased.* The karanga has a plaintive, repetitive melody, often compared to a *keening* or *pihe*. It's done in a call-and-response style between the host and visiting women, creating a *thread of sound* across the open courtyard of the marae. This sound is the very voice of grief and love, and it is said to guide the spirit as well: *"I was told that the main reason our people were so spiritual was because the spirits of the dead passed through our valley on the way to Te Ara Wairua... It was our job to help guide them through,"* recounted one Māori elder. Indeed, in one community, a blind elder would sit in his house constantly reciting *karakia* (prayers) to keep the spirits moving along the Spirits' Trail. We see here an explicit recognition that *rhythmic prayer and chant keep the flow of spirits orderly*—a duty very much akin to a continuous heartbeat of spirituality maintained for those in transition.

Throughout the tangi, *speech and song alternate in a structured rhythm*. Māori protocol dictates that when someone gives a *whaikōrero* (funeral oration), that speech is followed by a *waiata* (song) from the speaker's group. These waiata tangi (lament songs) are often ancient chants or hymns delivered in unison. One classic waiata tangi, *"Pō pō, e tangi ana tama ki te kai māna"* ("In the night, a child cries for food"), uses metaphor to express grief and is intoned in a slow, falling melody that many Māori say *"makes the heart weep."* The collective singing provides an emotional release and also a *collective breathing*—literally, as the group sings, their breaths and heartbeats can synchronize. Ethnographers note that these laments serve to *"express grief and connect the deceased with their iwi (tribe) and land." This connection to land is crucial: often, during tangi, speakers will recall the deceased's connection to specific mountains, rivers, and marae, essentially *"binding their heart back to the land"* in words.

The *haka*, a vigorous group dance with shouted chant, is another rhythmic element used in Māori farewells. There are special *funeral haka* (distinct from war haka) that embody profound respect and emotion. For example, when a great chief dies, warriors might perform a *Haka Taparahi* with loud *haka peruperu* style stomps and chants, not in aggression but in passionate honor. The unified stomping is like a communal heartbeat shaking the earth for the one who has passed, a final show of strength and love. One modern example widely seen was the haka performed by New Zealand soldiers at a comrade's funeral: they stomped and cried in unison, faces contorted in grief, channeling sorrow into fierce energy—this video went viral because it was so raw and powerful. It illustrated how the haka's *rhythm (slapping thighs, pounding chests, synchronized calls)* serves as an outlet for grief and a message to the spirit world that a great one is coming. The use of haka at tangi shows that for Māori, *emotion is given form through bodily rhythm*—whether that emotion is sorrow, love, or even humor (sometimes a light-hearted song is sung at the end of tangi to lift spirits, acknowledging life goes on).

After the burial, Māori observe additional rituals like the *hakari* (feast) and *whakanoa* (cleansing) to lift the tapu (sacred restriction) of mourning. Even these have rhythmic elements: the *clapping of hands* in prayer before the meal, the chants said by a tohunga (priest) as he sprinkles water to remove tapu. The entire process of tangihanga is thus enveloped in layers of sound and action that move in time.

For an outside observer or a practitioner, Māori death practices demonstrate the importance of *community performance* in processing death. The communal heartbeat is externalized: sometimes softly (in karanga and waiata), sometimes forcefully (in haka), but always collectively. There is a Māori proverb: *"He kōrero, he waiata, ka ora ai te iwi"*—"Through speech and song, the people thrive." At tangi, one might say, through speech and song, the people *survive* the immediate shock of loss, and the spirit is sent on.

In meditative or therapeutic adaptation, one might incorporate Māori elements by allowing (or even prompting) the family to perform familiar practices at the bedside. For instance, letting a Māori family sing a beloved hymn or waiata while their dying relative engages in relaxed breathing could be more comforting than silence. If appropriate, the facilitator might quietly count or tap in time with that song—creating a subtle unity of heartbeat and music. Visualizations can also draw on Māori cosmology: e.g., inviting a patient to imagine standing at Cape Reinga with ancestors beckoning from across the water, each heartbeat a *footstep toward a reunion* in Hawaiki. For Māori clients, acknowledging the presence of *whānau* (family) and *tipuna* (ancestors) can validate their experience. Even encouraging gentle *humming or chanting* during a session (if the person is comfortable) could tap into the deep Polynesian tradition of using voice as medicine.

The continent of Africa contains a vast tapestry of cultures, but many sub-Saharan African traditions share certain themes in their approach to death: a strong veneration of *ancestors*, the use of *drumming and music* to communicate and transform energy, and communal ceremonies that both mourn and celebrate. An oft-cited proverb from Ghana says, *"A funeral drum sounds in the distance for the death of a neighbor, and each beat of that drum beats within our own hearts."* This speaks to the communal nature of African life—one person's death reverberates through the community like a drumbeat.

In many African societies, the *drum is more than an instrument*—it is the voice of the community and a conduit to the spirit world. It has been said that "traditionally the drum was the heartbeat and soul of African communities...accompanying religious rites and rituals that call up ancestral spirits. Nowhere is this more evident than in African funeral ceremonies. For example, among the Ashanti people of West Africa (in present-day Ghana), funerals are multi-day events often held on specific days of the week (with Saturday being common for final funerals).

The Ashanti incorporate the use of *"talking drums"*—drums capable of imitating the tone and prosody of speech—to announce the news of death and to extol the deeds of the departed. Through skillful drumming, messages are conveyed in proverbial language. The drum might literally "speak" a phrase like *"A great tree has fallen in the forest"* to signify the passing of a respected elder. These rhythms both inform and unite the community in a shared experience of loss.

Once the funeral gathering convenes, music and dance become central. In Ashanti culture, as one ethnographer describes, *"these events are marked by traditional music, especially talking drums, which convey stories of the deceased's life and their passage to the afterlife. Drummed rhythms can recount ancient tales of death and the passage to the next world, adding a spiritual dimension to the event." The drummers will play patterns associated with mourning— often slower, with deep resonant beats like a somber heartbeat—and also more celebratory pieces that prompt people to dance. It is not unusual at Ashanti funerals to see mourners first weeping in a dirge and later dancing vigorously, clad in black and red funeral cloth, as a band plays highlife or traditional songs. This reflects the Ashanti view that funerals are *both a farewell and a celebration*—the person is being mourned and also properly sent off with honor and joy to join the ancestors. As one observer noted, *"Ashanti funerals blend solemnity with celebration, honoring both the life lived and the ancestral role the deceased will now play."

Throughout West and Central Africa, many cultures believe that the boundary between the living and the dead is thin. The dead become *ancestors* (*living-dead*, as Kenyan theologian John Mbiti called them) who actively influence and protect the living. Thus, death rituals aim to ensure a safe arrival into ancestorhood. In Nigeria, for example, the Yoruba people hold elaborate funeral ceremonies, especially for elders. These include nights of drumming, *àrokò* (chanting of praise-poems or oríkì for the deceased), and sometimes trance-possession dances where it is believed an ancestor's spirit may temporarily inhabit a dancer's body to give messages or blessings. The steady beat of the *bàtá drums* in Yoruba funerals is thought to please the *orishas* (divine spirits) and call the spirit of the deceased to join the realm of the revered ancestors. We see here a use of *rhythm as invocation*—much as MHbT uses rhythm to induce a meditative state, Yoruba drummers use it to induce a spiritual state in funeral participants, opening them to a connection with the beyond.

In East Africa, among the Luo of Kenya, funerals (tero buru) traditionally included dramatic displays of grief: loud wailing, *horn-blowing and drum-beating*, and even ceremonial mock attacks on the homestead by spear-wielding mourners to "fight off" death. The community might engage in nightly singing of *dirges* (*ohangla* songs) that have specific repetitive refrains, creating a hypnotic, heart-entraining effect on listeners. Elders would recite genealogies of the deceased with rhythmic emphasis, reinforcing the person's place in the chain of ancestors and ensuring their name "keeps beating" in the community's memory.

In Southern Africa, Zulu and Xhosa peoples similarly have rich funeral traditions. After Christian influence, many now sing *church hymns* at funerals—but often adapted into *call-and-response* patterns with African harmonies and drumming on hymn boards. In rural Zululand, for instance, it's common at night during the *ukubuyisa* (bringing home the spirit) ceremony to sing *izihlabelelo* (Christian hymns) in a low, cyclic manner around a fire. Meanwhile, a drum or even just clapping might keep time, giving a clear rhythm. One frequently sung Xhosa hymn at funerals is *"Lizalis' idinga lakho"* ("Fulfill Your Promise, Lord")—it starts slow and somber, then often quickens to a hand-clapping, swaying chorus. This shift in tempo can lead the mourners from tears to a kind of *spiritual high*, reflecting a therapeutic transformation of mood through music.

What ties these varied African examples together is the *role of rhythmic communal activity*. Whether through drum, song, or dance, the community creates a shared heartbeat to carry them through the loss. *"Traditionally, the drum was the heartbeat, the soul of most African communities."* This statement is no abstraction; at a funeral, when the communal drum is sounded, everyone's heart seems to synchronize to it. It provides a sense of unity and catharsis: in Ghana, for instance, women may form circles to perform *Adowa*, a slow, expressive funeral dance, moving their arms in time to the talking drum's story of the deceased's virtues. The dance has its own heartbeat—the stamping of feet and gentle clap at certain points. Men might fire rifles into the air three times (a loud percussion marking stages of the funeral). These auditory and kinetic rhythms help structure grief and give mourners roles to perform.

For a therapeutic setting, African traditions remind us that *embodied rhythm and collective expression can be deeply healing*. A patient from an African background might feel isolated in a quiet hospital room; integrating elements like gentle drumming or familiar spiritual songs could reconnect them to their cultural coping mechanisms. Even something as simple as playing a recording of traditional drums or choir songs quietly can provide comfort. Involving family in rhythmic activities—for example, encouraging them to gently tap or stroke the patient's hand in time with a hymn they hum—can allow the family's "heartbeat" to envelop the patient. A Zulu proverb says *"Umuntu ngumuntu ngabantu"* (a person is a person through other people). In death, too, an individual's heart is kept strong through the community's heartbeat. Recognizing this can guide practitioners to facilitate *group-centered* moments (like gathering family to sing the patient's favorite chorus in unison, rather than maintaining a medical silence).

In summary, the global indigenous perspectives from the Andes, Māori New Zealand, and Africa highlight a view of dying as a *ritual process embedded in community and nature*. They utilize the fundamental human tools of rhythm—drumming, chanting, singing, dancing, breathing—to navigate the mystery of death. These cultures remind us that the act of dying is not merely a medical event but a *social and spiritual event*, one that can be choreographed with culturally meaningful "heartbeats" so that the individual and the community find continuity and solace. For those of us in modern care roles, integrating these lessons—inviting the drum, the song, the ancestor invocation into the care plan—can lead to a more holistic and respectful support for patients from these backgrounds. It ensures that the final beats of their life's song are in harmony with the ancestral and cosmic music that has surrounded them all along.

COMMON THREADS AND THE
INTEGRATION OF CULTURAL RHYTHMS IN MHBT

Having journeyed through Native American, Buddhist, Christian, Jewish, and various Indigenous worldviews, we find remarkable commonalities amid the contrasts. Nearly every tradition envisions *death as a transition or journey*, not a mere end. Whether conceptualized as the soul traveling to an ancestral realm, the consciousness navigating a bardo, the spirit leaping to a homeland, or the individual awaiting resurrection, there is a shared understanding that something of the person—call it heart, soul, mind-stream, or legacy—carries on.

Across cultures, the *heart* stands as a potent symbol of this continuity. In biological fact, the heart's last beat marks clinical death. But spiritually, many peoples see the heart as containing the essence of a person. Ancient Egyptians weighed it against truth to judge the soul. Plains Indians called the drumbeat the Great Spirit's heart, aligning human hearts with the land's. The Bible speaks of *"creating a pure heart"* and *"hardening hearts,"* implying the heart's moral and spiritual centrality. We saw in Christianity the Sacred Heart devotion and We saw in Buddhism the practice of placing the mind in the heart at death. In countless funeral songs and eulogies worldwide, the heart is invoked—*"my heart will go on," "our hearts are broken,"* etc. The metaphor of the heart as the seat of life and love is virtually universal. For a modality like Meditative Heartbeat Therapy, this is a validating insight: focusing on the heartbeat as a bridge between life and death resonates deeply with human cultural heritage. It taps into a primal understanding that the *heart's rhythm is the rhythm of life*, and aligning with it can open pathways of meaning and connection.

Another common thread is the use of *rhythm, music, and breath* to sanctify and ease the dying process. Around the world, people chant or sing at the bedside of the dying. This may take the form of monks reciting sutras in a measured tone, a priest intoning prayers, family members singing a favorite hymn, or villagers drumming and dancing. These acts are not mere art; they serve profound psychological and spiritual purposes. Rhythmic sound can entrain breathing—as seen when a group's singing calms a patient's respirations and heartbeat. Music can trigger memory, emotion, and transcendence—a final hymn might bring a dying person to peaceful tears and acceptance. In many traditions, specific rhythms are believed to literally guide the soul: the Pure Land Buddhist believes continuous chanting of Amitābha's name forms a kind of sound current to the Pure Land; the African drummer believes his drum calls the ancestors to carry the soul home; the Navajo singer's chant restores cosmic order (hozho) so the soul departs unconfused.

The *breath* is also central in several practices. The Hebrew term *neshamah* (soul) is linked to *neshima* (breath); the Greek *pneuma* and Sanskrit *prāna* similarly mean spirit-breath. Many cultures have understood death as the moment the breath (life-spirit) leaves the body—hence the English "expire" (exhale) for dying. It is common that when the last breath occurs, those present become very still, and then perform ritual actions: in Catholicism, the priest might pray *"Go forth, O soul"; in Hinduism, family might whisper *"Rama"* in the ear at the final breath; in Buddhism, they do not disturb the body for a while to allow subtle breathing to cease. This universality of attending to the breath at death underscores how focusing on breath in therapy (a key part of mindfulness and MHbT) is culturally appropriate across many contexts. The idea of *"breathing out"* pain or *"breathing in"* peace can be explained in religious terms if needed (e.g. to a Christian: "receive the Holy Spirit on each inhale, release your burden on each exhale," echoing John 20:22).

We also see a common thread of the *community's role*. Few traditions expect people to die alone. From the Jewish mitzvah of accompanying the dying, to the Irish wake, to the constant presence at a Māori tangi, there is an implicit understanding that the *community forms a circle of support* at life's end. This community often acts in rhythmic unity—chanting together, praying responsively, singing in harmony, dancing in sync. It's as if the community provides an external heartbeat when the individual's own is faltering. Indeed, in a literal sense, when others hold or embrace the dying, or even place a hand on their chest, their hearts may beat together for those last moments. This communal aspect suggests that in modern care, we should invite and facilitate family participation whenever possible. Their *voices and touches* are not distractions but can be central to the patient's spiritual comfort.

While commonalities abound, we also must respect differences. For instance, while one culture may want exuberant drumming, another may insist on quiet solemnity. Spiritual integration is not one-size-fits-all. The key is to *ask and listen*: What does the patient find meaningful? Who or what do they want present? Many times, patients will draw on their heritage if given the chance. Our role is often to *give permission* or enable logistics for these cultural expressions. A hospital might be an alien environment for a family to conduct a ritual, but a sensitive practitioner can advocate: e.g., allowing a small *electric candle* in the ICU for a vigil, or permitting a *hand drum or rattle* in a hospice even if it's unusual.

From the perspective of Meditative Heartbeat Therapy (MHbT), these cultural insights enrich the practice. MHbT already uses the *universal language of the heartbeat* and breathing. By overlaying culturally resonant elements—be it phrases, imagery, or sounds—the therapy becomes not just calming but *personally meaningful*. For example:

- With a Navajo patient, one might incorporate the concept of *hozho* (harmony) by having them visualize their heartbeat aligning with the "heartbeat" of the universe, restoring balance (much like their chants aim to do).
- With a Catholic patient, one might suggest each heartbeat is echoed by the Sacred Heart of Jesus, or time the Jesus Prayer to the pulse.
- With a Chinese Buddhist, one might synchronize a mantra

chant (even if whispered) to the heart's rhythm, recalling how Pure Land adepts recite "*Amituofo.*"

- With an Ashanti patient, one could play a recording of *talking drum* rhythms softly and invite them to relax into that ancestral sound as they focus on their own heart—thus feeling enveloped by the community's heartbeat even if far from home.

Finally, all these traditions underscore that *the end of life can be a time of deep meaning and even beauty*, not only sorrow. There is a reason so many rituals involve *color, song, incense, story*. They are trying to elevate the moment beyond the mundane, to mark the significance of the transition. In our contemporary approach, we too can help elevate the dying experience by bringing in these elements in an appropriate way. Rather than a sterile, purely clinical event, death can once again become a rich human event—one in which the dying person feels connected to something larger: be it God, ancestors, nature, or community.

As we integrate cultural diversity in spiritual end-of-life care, we ultimately reaffirm a simple truth: *every human heart beats to the rhythm of a story*. That story may be told through drums or prayers or lullabies, but at its core it is the story of our connection—to each other and to the mystery beyond. Meditative Heartbeat Therapy, by literally tuning into the heartbeat, provides a natural platform for these stories to be honored. By listening to the heart, we listen to the life it encapsulated.

In closing, let us recall the image of a circle of people around a dying individual—be it a family singing a gentle song, monks chanting *Om mani padme hum*, friends drumming a slow cadence, or nurses and chaplains quietly praying. In all these scenes, there is a palpable shared heartbeat of compassion. Our task is to *join that circle*, to add our voice or drum or silent presence to that rhythm, and to help the one at the center feel carried by it. As the final breath comes and the physical heart falls silent, the *spiritual heartbeat*—kept by the living and, many believe, joined by the ancestors—continues.

In that continued rhythm, the dying find their place in the eternal song.

Such is the power of integrating cultural rhythms and heart-centered practices at the end of life: it helps ensure that when a person's final moment arrives, they do not walk that path in silence, but *accompanied by the heartbeat of those who love them, the echoes of those who came before, and the promise that life's melody goes on.*

REFLECTION

THE POWER OF STORIES IN
HEALING AND TRANSFORMATION

When we encounter the stories of others, we do more than simply absorb their experiences. We connect with the essence of their lives—their struggles, triumphs, fears, and hopes. These stories invite us to see beyond the surface and to witness the intricacies of human existence, revealing the rich tapestry of emotions and experiences that shape us all. Through the stories shared in the practice of Meditative Heartbeat Therapy (MHbT), we learn not only about others but also about ourselves.

These stories serve as mirrors, reflecting our own journey of healing and transformation. They remind us that healing is not a linear process—it is a fluid, often unpredictable experience. We may go into a healing process with clear intentions, seeking relief from pain or fear, yet find that healing takes shape in ways we did not anticipate. Some of the most profound moments of healing occur in silence, in connection, in acceptance. These stories teach us that the process of becoming whole is as diverse as the individuals who seek it, and it is often shaped by forces we cannot control or predict.

Healing is not confined to specific outcomes—it is about being present to whatever emerges. Each heartbeat, each person's journey, speaks to a different truth. And it is in the stories of others that we begin to see how the heartbeat, though unique to every individual, is a thread that connects us all in the shared human experience.

The stories of those who engage in MHbT are not isolated; they serve as bridges connecting the deeply personal to the universal. Grief, fear, hope, and love—these are not private emotions but shared experiences that resonate across the human condition. When we listen to these stories, we find echoes of our own lives in the experiences of others. Through the lens of empathy, we see how interconnected we all are, how our struggles and joys are woven together in the vast fabric of human existence.

Empathy is not simply a passive feeling—it is an active practice. It involves stepping into another's story, feeling their emotions, and understanding their reality. MHbT allows us to do this not only through words but through presence. When we listen to someone else's heartbeat, we are listening to their story in its most intimate form. The rhythm of their heart becomes the language of their experience, a silent conversation that transcends words and connects us at the deepest level.

In this way, each session of MHbT is an opportunity to practice empathy—not just as an abstract concept, but as a lived, embodied act. To listen to the heartbeat is to listen with the heart, to feel another's journey as if it were our own, and to honor their experience as part of our shared human path.

The stories shared through MHbT teach us that healing is rarely simple or straightforward. It often unfolds in unexpected ways, offering insights and transformations that cannot be predicted. A patient may begin a session seeking relief from anxiety, only to find themselves unexpectedly confronting unresolved emotions or memories long buried. A family may come together with the hope of finding closure, only to discover a deeper connection with their loved one in the final moments of life.

These stories illuminate the complexity of healing—it is not always about achieving a specific outcome or reaching a final destination. Rather, it is about creating space for whatever needs to emerge in the moment. Sometimes healing manifests as acceptance, sometimes as reconciliation, and sometimes as a shift in perspective that renews the sense of purpose. MHbT encourages us to approach healing with an open heart, free from expectations, and to listen attentively to the lessons that each moment offers.

This openness allows for transformation to occur, even in the most unexpected ways. The heartbeat teaches us that healing is a dynamic process, one that is shaped by the rhythms of life itself. It invites us to trust the journey, knowing that sometimes the most profound shifts happen when we least expect them.

At the heart of every healing story is vulnerability—a willingness to face the unknown, to sit with discomfort, and to open ourselves to the possibility of transformation. Vulnerability is often seen as a weakness, but in the context of MHbT, it becomes a gateway to healing. It takes courage to be vulnerable, to sit with difficult emotions, and to listen to the heart without turning away. Yet, it is precisely in these moments of vulnerability that profound transformation occurs.

When patients and caregivers allow themselves to be vulnerable —whether by confronting fears, expressing unspoken emotions, or simply allowing themselves to feel—they open the door to connection. This connection is not limited to others; it also extends inward, creating a deeper relationship with the self. Vulnerability invites us to embrace all parts of ourselves—the fears, the joys, the uncertainties —and to approach healing with acceptance rather than resistance.

MHbT creates a safe space for vulnerability, where individuals are encouraged to explore their emotions without judgment. It reminds us that vulnerability is not something to be feared or avoided, but rather something to be welcomed as a powerful tool for growth. In these moments of openness, we come into deeper contact with our own humanity, and in doing so, we find the potential for true healing.

One of the most transformative aspects of MHbT is the role it plays in family healing. The act of listening to a loved one's heartbeat creates a powerful space for connection, where words are not necessary. This shared experience transcends the boundaries of language, allowing family members to express love, presence, and support in ways that go beyond what they may be able to articulate.

For families facing the end of life, this shared ritual becomes a moment of profound intimacy. Tensions that may have existed for years can dissolve in the presence of the heartbeat, replaced by a deep sense of unity and peace. Family members are given the opportunity to express love and connection, sometimes for the first time, in a space where the focus is not on fixing or resolving, but on simply being present with one another.

MHbT shifts the focus of caregiving from symptom management to relational connection. It teaches us that healing occurs not just in isolation but in relationships. By creating a space for presence and love, MHbT fosters a deeper understanding of what it means to care for one another—not through solutions or fixes, but through genuine connection and shared experience.

The stories shared through MHbT often extend beyond the physical realm of life and death. The heartbeat, once a symbol of life, becomes a lasting legacy—a rhythm that continues to echo long after a person has passed. Some families choose to keep recordings of a loved one's heartbeat, integrating them into personal rituals or memorial services as a way of keeping the connection alive. These recordings become more than just mementos; they become an embodiment of the love and presence that remain after a person's physical form is gone.

In this way, the heartbeat carries the essence of the person forward, extending beyond the boundaries of life itself. It is a reminder that connection does not end with death but continues in the rhythms we carry with us. Each time we listen to the heartbeat—whether our own or someone else's—we are reminded of the lasting impact we have on one another, and of the interconnectedness that transcends time and space.

Caregivers, too, benefit from the lessons of MHbT. Often burdened by exhaustion and emotional fatigue, caregivers can find themselves disconnected from their own needs. MHbT offers them a way to reconnect with themselves through the practice of presence.

By listening to the heartbeat, caregivers are reminded of their own humanity—their own need for care, rest, and connection.

This act of listening becomes a form of self-care, grounding caregivers in the rhythm of life and reminding them that they are not alone in their work. It teaches them that caregiving is not about carrying the burden of others' pain in isolation but about creating spaces of connection, for themselves as well as for others. In this way, MHbT offers caregivers the opportunity to care for their own hearts, fostering balance between the act of giving and the act of receiving.

One of the most profound realizations offered by MHbT is the universality of the heartbeat. Regardless of our background, culture, or individual story, we all share the same rhythm. The heartbeat is a symbol of the pulse of life itself, a reminder that, at our core, we are all connected. It is through this shared rhythm that we understand the interconnectedness of all beings, and it is in this connection that we find solace and strength.

In listening to the heartbeat, we acknowledge our shared humanity. We recognize that, despite our differences, we are all part of the same rhythm—a rhythm that transcends the individual and unites us in the broader story of life. This awareness fosters empathy and compassion, reminding us that we are never truly alone, even in our most difficult moments.

As we move forward from the case studies shared in MHbT, let us carry these stories with us. Let us remember that healing is not solely about outcomes but about presence—about being fully with ourselves and others in every moment. Let us embrace the lessons of vulnerability, connection, and empathy, knowing that these are the rhythms that guide us through life.

Take a moment now to place your hand over your heart. Feel the rhythm beneath your palm. In this rhythm, there is a reminder: you are not alone. Your story is part of a larger story—one that is written in the rhythm of the heartbeat, one that continues beyond this moment, beyond this life.

Let each story become a heartbeat—a rhythm that carries you forward, one beat at a time.

Let these stories remind you of the power of presence, the importance of connection, and the beauty of living fully, even in the face of uncertainty. And as you listen to your own heartbeat, know that you are part of this rhythm—a rhythm that unites us all, across time, space, and experience.

PART THREE
CLINICAL APPLICATIONS

This section offers a detailed exploration of Meditative Heartbeat Therapy in action. Building on its spiritual and philosophical foundations, we now turn to the bedside, where sound, breath, and presence converge in real clinical settings. These chapters present practical applications of MHbT across a range of palliative care experiences: from the gentle regulation of emotional distress to its integration with supplemental oxygen, from sacred ritual to sound-supported hypnosis, from culturally inclusive care to the intimate accompaniment of end-of-life doulas. Through each application, MHbT remains rooted in its core mission—to restore meaning, dignity, and connection in the final days of life. Whether you are a clinician, chaplain, caregiver, or doula, this section is your guide to practicing MHbT with intention and reverence.

CHAPTER 9

INTEGRATIVE PALLIATIVE CARE AND MHBT

I ntegrative palliative care represents a holistic and patient-centered approach to managing the complex needs of individuals facing serious or terminal illnesses. By combining conventional medical treatments with evidence-based integrative therapies, this model seeks to alleviate physical symptoms while also addressing emotional, psychological, and spiritual distress. In this landscape, Meditative Heartbeat Therapy (MHbT) emerges as a groundbreaking modality that enhances traditional palliative care methods by uniquely harnessing the rhythm of a patient's own heartbeat to foster deep relaxation, connection, and healing.

Palliative care has traditionally focused on relieving suffering and improving quality of life for patients with life-threatening conditions. The field emerged as a response to the limitations of curative medical interventions, emphasizing comfort and dignity in the face of illness. While modern palliative care remains rooted in symptom management and supportive care, the integration of complementary therapies has expanded its scope, providing patients with a more holistic approach to healing.

The rise of integrative palliative care can be attributed to several factors:

1. *Patient Demand*—As awareness of alternative healing methods grows, many patients express interest in non-pharmacological interventions for symptom relief.
2. *Scientific Validation*—A growing body of research supports the efficacy of integrative therapies such as meditation, music therapy, guided imagery, and energy healing in palliative care.
3. *Personalized Medicine Movement*—Modern healthcare increasingly values patient-centered approaches that consider individual preferences, values, and holistic well-being.
4. *Healthcare System Challenges*—Overreliance on pharmaceuticals for symptom management has led to concerns over polypharmacy, side effects, and limited effectiveness in addressing emotional and spiritual distress.

By incorporating integrative therapies into palliative care, clinicians can offer a more balanced approach to managing pain, anxiety, fatigue, and existential suffering.

Integrative palliative care is guided by several key principles:

- *Whole-Person Care:* Recognizing that patients are more than their disease, this approach seeks to address physical, emotional, social, and spiritual needs.
- *Personalization:* Treatment plans are tailored to individual patient preferences and cultural backgrounds.
- *Evidence-Based Integration:* While incorporating diverse healing modalities, integrative palliative care relies on therapies that have demonstrated efficacy in clinical settings.
- *Collaboration Across Disciplines:* A multidisciplinary team approach ensures that patients receive comprehensive care, blending the expertise of physicians, nurses, chaplains, social workers, and integrative therapists.

- *Enhancing Quality of Life:* The ultimate goal is to promote comfort, peace, and meaning in the patient's remaining time, regardless of prognosis.

MHbT aligns seamlessly with these principles by offering a deeply personal and non-invasive intervention that fosters inner calm, presence, and connection.

MHbT is a unique mind-body therapy that utilizes the rhythmic sound of a patient's own heartbeat as the focal point of meditation. This practice draws upon several key mechanisms:

- *Interoceptive Awareness:* By attuning to the natural rhythm of the heart, patients develop a heightened awareness of their internal states, fostering self-regulation and emotional resilience.
- *Neurosensory Entrainment:* The repetition of a familiar and intrinsic sound (one's own heartbeat) can induce a deeply meditative state, slowing brain wave activity and promoting relaxation.
- *Biofeedback and Self-Soothing:* Unlike external music or guided meditations, the use of one's own heartbeat creates an intimate and self-generated method of comfort and grounding.

As an independent intervention, MHbT offers several benefits that distinguish it from other integrative therapies:

- *Highly Personalized:* Unlike generic meditation recordings or pre-designed relaxation tracks, MHbT is inherently unique to each patient, making it deeply meaningful.
- *Accessible and Non-Invasive:* Patients can engage in MHbT regardless of physical condition, cognitive capacity, or level of consciousness, making it an inclusive therapy for all stages of illness.

- *Promotes Emotional Processing:* The steady, rhythmic nature of heartbeat-based meditation allows patients to engage in deep reflection, making it useful for processing grief, existential distress, and unresolved emotions.

MHbT can be seamlessly integrated with a variety of other therapeutic modalities:

- *Clinical Hypnosis:* MHbT enhances the effects of hypnosis by providing an intrinsic auditory anchor, helping patients achieve deeper states of trance and relaxation.
- *Mindfulness and Meditation Practices:* The heartbeat serves as a natural object of focus, reinforcing mindfulness principles of present-moment awareness and non-judgmental observation.
- *Music Therapy:* When incorporated into personalized musical compositions, the recorded heartbeat can create an emotionally resonant and soothing auditory experience.
- *Guided Imagery and Visualization:* Patients can synchronize visualization exercises with the rhythm of their heartbeat, deepening the immersive quality of these techniques.

CASE STUDY 1: MANAGING END-OF-LIFE ANXIETY

Mr. Thomas, a 72-year-old retired engineer, had been diagnosed with terminal lung cancer that had metastasized to his bones. The progression of the disease left him breathless, frail, and increasingly dependent on his caregivers. Along with the physical toll, he was grappling with severe anxiety, particularly as his life drew to a close. His anxiety manifested in constant restlessness, nightmares, difficulty breathing, and an overwhelming sense of impending doom. Despite being on a high dose of anxiolytics, including benzodiazepines, his symptoms persisted, and he experienced significant emotional and existential distress.

MHbT was introduced in conjunction with clinical hypnosis as part of an integrative palliative care plan. The therapist began with gentle body awareness techniques, guiding Mr. Thomas to focus on his breath before incorporating his own heartbeat as a grounding tool. A recorded heartbeat, obtained through a biofeedback device, was used as the main auditory anchor in his sessions. This allowed Mr. Thomas to center his awareness on the steady, rhythmic sound of his own heartbeat, which was soothing and deeply personal.

Alongside this, clinical hypnosis was used to deepen his state of relaxation. During these sessions, the therapist led Mr. Thomas through a series of guided visualizations aimed at helping him accept his mortality and create a sense of inner peace. He was guided to visualize himself floating in a peaceful, safe space, accompanied by the steady beat of his heart, which he was asked to sync with his breathing.

After two weeks of daily MHbT sessions, Mr. Thomas began to experience profound shifts in his anxiety levels. He reported that the rhythmic sound of his heartbeat was both comforting and grounding, offering a connection to his body that felt reassuring during moments of distress. In one instance, he recalled a particularly anxious night when, instead of reaching for his anxiety medication, he chose to focus on the sound of his heartbeat, breathing deeply in sync with it. Within 20 minutes, his anxiety lessened, and he was able to sleep without medication.

As the therapy continued, Mr. Thomas gradually reduced his use of sedative medications, which had previously been his primary means of coping. He also began to report a significant decrease in feelings of panic and dread. His caregivers noted that his increased ability to find calm allowed him to be more present in his final days, engaging in meaningful conversations with his family and reflecting on his life with a sense of peace.

This case exemplifies the potential of MHbT to manage anxiety and provide emotional and psychological relief for patients facing terminal illness. By leveraging the deeply personal and soothing sound of one's own heartbeat, MHbT helped Mr. Thomas find a sense of tranquility, even in the face of his imminent death. The integration of clinical hypnosis further amplified the effectiveness of MHbT, offering a multi-layered approach to managing end-of-life anxiety.

CASE STUDY 2:
ENHANCING COMFORT IN ADVANCED DEMENTIA

Mrs. Evelyn, an 84-year-old woman, had been diagnosed with advanced Alzheimer's disease. Over the course of her illness, she had become progressively more agitated, particularly in the late afternoon and evening, a condition known as "sundowning." She would frequently become disoriented, expressing confusion, anxiety, and aggression toward her caregivers. She struggled to recognize family members and would often exhibit repetitive behaviors and vocalizations. Traditional approaches, including pharmacological interventions, were only partially effective in managing her symptoms. The family and caregivers were concerned about her quality of life and sought alternative, non-pharmacological methods to reduce her agitation and provide comfort.

The hospice team introduced MHbT as part of a holistic care plan, working alongside music therapy. The therapist played a recorded version of Mrs. Evelyn's heartbeat, which was paired with gentle instrumental music that she had enjoyed in her younger years. The rhythmic pulse of her heartbeat, combined with the soft melodies, created an auditory landscape that felt familiar and soothing. The sessions were conducted in a calm, quiet room with soft lighting, promoting a peaceful environment that helped reduce overstimulation.

The therapist began each session by gently guiding Mrs. Evelyn's attention to the sound of her heartbeat. She was encouraged to focus on the sensation of her breath moving in time with the beat, helping her regulate her breathing and bring her attention away from agitation. The music was designed to be simple and repetitive, further reinforcing the calming effects of the heartbeat and providing a sense of emotional safety.

Over the course of several weeks, the hospice team noticed significant improvements in Mrs. Evelyn's mood and behavior. Her episodes of agitation decreased dramatically, with her family reporting fewer instances of outbursts and distress. During the times when she became upset or confused, the caregivers would play the heartbeat recording and music, which provided an immediate calming effect. Mrs. Evelyn began to recognize the sound of her heartbeat and seemed comforted by its presence, even during moments of disorientation.

Her physical state also improved; she began to regulate her breathing more effectively and showed a reduction in the hyperventilation episodes that were previously common. This, in turn, helped her caregivers manage her symptoms more effectively, as she required fewer interventions to calm down. The use of MHbT provided Mrs. Evelyn with a sense of security and connection, even as cognitive decline continued.

This case underscores the power of MHbT to provide emotional and physiological regulation for patients with advanced dementia. By using a deeply personal, soothing auditory stimulus, such as the recorded heartbeat, and pairing it with music therapy, the intervention created a non-invasive and highly effective means of managing agitation and promoting relaxation. MHbT was not only a tool for symptom management but also a means of fostering a sense of emotional connection and comfort in a patient who had difficulty recognizing others.

CASE STUDY 3: MHBT IN PEDIATRIC PALLIATIVE CARE

Sophia, a 9-year-old girl, had been diagnosed with a rare and progressive neurological disorder that caused her to experience chronic, severe pain and debilitating muscle spasms. Despite trying numerous medications, including opioids, to manage her symptoms, she continued to experience persistent pain, which greatly impacted her ability to sleep, engage in daily activities, and maintain a positive outlook. Her parents were concerned about the long-term effects of opioid use and sought alternative methods to manage her pain and improve her quality of life.

Sophia's care team introduced MHbT as part of a multi-modal pain management strategy. Her recorded heartbeat was paired with a guided meditation that involved focusing on the rhythmic sound while visualizing a peaceful landscape. The therapist tailored the visualization to Sophia's interests, incorporating images of a beautiful meadow filled with flowers and gentle breezes. The therapist used imagery of Sophia's heartbeat gently syncing with the rhythm of the natural environment, helping her to feel connected to the soothing flow of life.

During the sessions, Sophia was guided to use the heartbeat as an anchor whenever she felt pain or discomfort, helping her focus on something familiar and calming rather than the sensation of pain. The therapist also introduced slow breathing exercises, encouraging Sophia to breathe deeply in sync with her heartbeat, helping to activate the parasympathetic nervous system and reduce pain perception.

Within a week of starting MHbT sessions, Sophia began to experience notable improvements in both her sleep and pain levels. She reported feeling less pain when listening to her heartbeat and practicing deep breathing techniques. Her parents observed that she was able to fall asleep more easily and slept for longer periods, waking up feeling more rested and less irritable. Over the course of several weeks, Sophia's need for opioid pain medication decreased by approximately 30%, and she was able to manage her pain through more natural methods.

Sophia also became more engaged in daily activities, spending time with her family without being overwhelmed by pain. Her ability to participate in schoolwork and play increased, and her overall emotional well-being improved. She expressed a sense of control over her body, which helped her feel empowered in the face of her chronic illness.

This case demonstrates the versatility of MHbT in pediatric palliative care, offering a non-pharmacological option for managing chronic pain and improving sleep. By focusing on the natural rhythm of her heartbeat and pairing it with visualization techniques, Sophia found a therapeutic tool that allowed her to cope with pain in a more holistic and manageable way. MHbT not only helped reduce her reliance on medications but also improved her overall quality of life by fostering a sense of calm and empowerment.

CASE STUDY 4: SPIRITUAL REFLECTION IN HOSPICE CARE

Margaret, a 68-year-old woman with metastatic breast cancer, had entered hospice care after multiple rounds of chemotherapy and radiation proved ineffective. As she approached the end of her life, Margaret struggled with feelings of isolation, fear, and existential despair. Although she had been a devout spiritual person, she found it difficult to reconcile her beliefs with the suffering she was enduring. She expressed a desire for spiritual peace but was unsure how to achieve it in her final days.

MHbT was introduced as part of a comprehensive spiritual care plan. The therapist worked with Margaret to explore her life reflections through a guided meditation based on the rhythm of her heartbeat. Each session began with the sound of her heartbeat, followed by a gentle exploration of her life's key moments—her accomplishments, the love she had shared, and the people who had been most meaningful to her. The therapist encouraged Margaret to listen to the rhythm of her heart as a metaphor for the continuity of life, even in the face of physical decline.

Through guided visualization, Margaret was led to envision a spiritual transition, focusing on the rhythm of her heartbeat as a bridge between her physical life and the afterlife. The therapist emphasized the idea that the rhythm of her heart would continue even beyond her physical death, helping her embrace her mortality with peace and acceptance.

Margaret experienced profound spiritual healing as she engaged with the MHbT sessions. She reported a growing sense of inner peace and began to feel more connected to her faith, despite her physical decline. In one particularly moving session, she described experiencing a deep sense of connection to her late husband, whose heartbeat she could recall from their years together. This connection gave her a sense of closure, knowing that the rhythm of love and life was continuous.

Her anxiety about death decreased significantly, and she began to speak more openly with her family about her hopes for a peaceful transition. Margaret's final days were marked by a sense of tranquility that had eluded her in the earlier stages of her illness. She passed away peacefully, with her family by her side, after sharing a final meditation session that focused on the rhythmic pulse of her heart and the love that would endure.

This case illustrates the potential of MHbT to facilitate spiritual healing and provide a profound sense of closure for patients nearing the end of life. By connecting the rhythm of the heartbeat with life reflections and spiritual imagery, the therapy helped Margaret find peace with her impending death, transforming her final days into a deeply meaningful and spiritually fulfilling experience.

CASE STUDY 5: PTSD AND PALLIATIVE PATIENTS

John, a 64-year-old Vietnam War veteran, had been receiving palliative care for advanced liver disease caused by hepatitis C. He also suffered from severe post-traumatic stress disorder (PTSD), which had plagued him for decades. Flashbacks, nightmares, and heightened arousal were daily challenges for John, significantly affecting his physical and emotional well-being. His PTSD was compounded by the stress of his terminal illness, leading to feelings of helplessness, anxiety, and fear.

MHbT was introduced as a tool to help John manage his PTSD symptoms, particularly during moments of heightened anxiety or flashbacks. The therapist worked with John to focus on the rhythmic sound of his heartbeat as a grounding technique. By using the heartbeat as an anchor, John was encouraged to bring his attention away from traumatic memories and into the present moment.

In addition, the therapist incorporated mindfulness techniques, encouraging John to synchronize his breath with his heartbeat to activate the relaxation response. This combination of MHbT and mindfulness practices helped John shift from a state of hypervigilance to one of calm, allowing him to better regulate his emotional responses.

Within a few sessions, John began to notice significant reductions in the frequency and intensity of his flashbacks. The sound of his heartbeat became a reliable tool for bringing him back to the present moment whenever he felt overwhelmed by traumatic memories. His caregivers reported that he was able to engage more in conversations and spend time with his family without being consumed by anxiety.

John also experienced improvements in his sleep. He began to fall asleep more easily and stay asleep longer, without waking up in a panic. His PTSD symptoms, while not fully eliminated, were much more manageable, allowing him to experience a greater sense of peace as he neared the end of his life.

This case illustrates how MHbT can effectively address trauma-related distress in palliative care patients. By using the heartbeat as an anchor for grounding and mindfulness, the therapy helped John manage PTSD symptoms, leading to a more peaceful and emotionally stable end-of-life experience.

REFLECTION
THE RHYTHM THAT BINDS US

We enter this world carried by the rhythm of a heartbeat —not our own, but another's. Long before we take our first breath, before we open our eyes to the light of the world, we are cradled in the steady, unfaltering beat of the mother's heart. It is our first sound, our first comfort, our first proof that we belong to something beyond ourselves. In the quiet, dark sanctuary of the womb, we are tethered to life through rhythm.

And then, we are born, and with the first inhale, the first wail, we are met with a new rhythm—our own. Our heartbeat, now independent, carries us forward. It speeds with excitement, slows in sorrow, steadies in moments of peace. It plays its part in the great symphony of life, pulsing through our days unnoticed yet essential. We do not summon it, yet it is ours. We do not control it, yet it shapes the entirety of our experience.

In childhood, our heartbeat races as we run, wild and free, across fields of play. In youth, it quickens in love and longing, in anger and triumph, in fear and exhilaration. In the quiet hours of adulthood, it pulses with patience, with waiting, with endurance. And in the final stretch of life, it slows, like waves retreating from the shore, whispering of the great stillness to come.

The rhythm of the heart is more than a biological function; it is a sacred thread that binds us to the essence of life itself. Across time and culture, it has been honored as a sign of vitality, emotion, and the ineffable mystery of being alive. It is the first rhythm we know and the last one we surrender. And within it, we find an invitation—to return to ourselves, to listen, to be still, to know that even in suffering, there is something within us that remains steady, something whole and enduring.

For those at the threshold of life's great transition, the heartbeat becomes a final companion, a grounding presence when words no longer serve, when memory fades, when even breath itself grows weary. It is the last song of the body, and in its gentle cadence, we find a truth too profound for language.

To sit with a dying person is to witness the sacred in its most raw and unguarded form. We hold hands, we listen, we breathe together. In these moments, time itself shifts. The past dissolves, the future is irrelevant, and all that remains is the present—the steady pulse of life still flowing, still reaching, even in the midst of departure.

In the case studies we have explored, we see how Meditative Heartbeat Therapy serves as a bridge between fear and peace, between suffering and surrender. The anxious mind, caught in the tumult of uncertainty, learns to settle into its own familiar rhythm. The child in pain, too young to fully grasp what is happening, finds solace in the steady beat that reminds her she is still here. The elder, long adrift in the fog of dementia, is called back—if only for a while—by the sound of the life force still within her. The soldier, haunted by the echoes of war, finds grounding in the rhythm that has carried him through battles seen and unseen.

There is something profoundly human about recognizing our own heartbeat as a source of comfort. Unlike external music, unlike the words of another, the sound of our own life force reminds us that we are present. That even in suffering, we are whole. That even as the body prepares to let go, something within us still holds on.

Unitarian Universalist wisdom teaches that we are part of an interconnected web, that we do not move through this life alone. And yet, so often, we feel separate—adrift in our own pain, our own struggles, our own fear of the unknown. But within the heartbeat is a deeper truth: we are never truly alone.

What is the heartbeat, after all, but an echo of something greater? Our individual rhythm is not separate from the rhythms of the world. The tides rise and fall in their own steady cadence. The seasons move in a cycle, neither hurried nor delayed. The breath of the Earth itself, in the rustling of leaves, the pulsing of ocean waves, the migrations of birds, follows a rhythm older than time.

To listen to our own heartbeat is to remember that we belong to this greater rhythm. We are not isolated bodies moving toward an end. We are part of something vast, something ancient, something eternal. And when our individual rhythm fades, when the heart releases its final note, we do not vanish. We return. We merge with the greater pulse of existence, carried forward in ways beyond our knowing.

For those of us who remain, grief often brings a silence that feels unbearable. The absence of a beloved heartbeat—one we had listened to in hugs, in whispers, in nights of quiet breathing beside us —leaves a void. And yet, if we listen closely, if we become still enough, we may hear that their rhythm has not ceased. It has simply changed form. It has moved into the wind, into the rain, into the pulse of all things. They are not gone; they have only joined the larger song.

CHAPTER 10

INTEGRATING MHBT, REIKI, AND CLINICAL HYPNOSIS

I n palliative and end-of-life care, patients often grapple with *persistent pain and profound anxiety*, which can diminish their quality of life and strain their emotional well-being. While pharmacological treatments like opioids effectively address physical pain, they may leave *emotional, spiritual, and psychological dimensions* unresolved. Combining *Meditative Heartbeat Therapy (MHbT)*, *Reiki*, and *Clinical Hypnosis* offers an integrative and holistic method for alleviating pain and anxiety, enhancing both physical and emotional comfort.

- *MHbT* creates a steady *biological anchor*, allowing patients to focus on their heartbeat as a source of stability and calm.
- *Reiki* promotes energetic flow and relaxation, enabling patients to release physical and emotional tension.
- *Clinical Hypnosis* alters the patient's perception of pain, helping them access *subconscious resources* for relief and healing.

By addressing the *mind-body-spirit connection*, this integrative approach empowers patients to experience *greater ease, reduced suffering, and deeper emotional resilience.*

The heartbeat is uniquely positioned as both a *biological rhythm* and a *metaphorical representation* of life and connection. Its natural cadence resonates across multiple dimensions:

1. *Physiological Regulation:*
2. The steady rhythm of the heartbeat activates the parasympathetic nervous system, which counteracts the body's stress response and promotes relaxation.
3. *Emotional Grounding:*
4. Patients who focus on their heartbeat often find it easier to *regulate intense emotions*, breaking the cycle of pain-induced anxiety.
5. *Spiritual Connection:*
6. Many patients associate their heartbeat with their *essence or soul*, making it a powerful anchor for spiritual exploration and meaning-making.

Reiki complements MHbT by creating a state of *energetic harmony* that helps the patient relax and engage more fully with their therapeutic experience.

- *Energetic Release:* Reiki works to unblock areas of energetic stagnation that often correlate with physical pain or emotional distress.
- *Amplification of Calm:* The soothing nature of Reiki enhances the patient's ability to focus on their heartbeat, deepening their meditative state.

Clinical Hypnosis brings the *power of guided imagery and suggestion* to the integrated approach. By reframing pain as a manageable sensation or symbol, patients can regain a sense of control.

- *Pain as a Signal:* Hypnosis helps patients reinterpret pain as a *message from the body*, reducing fear and resistance.
- *Hypnotic Imagery:* Techniques like visualizing pain as a flame that dims with each heartbeat provide an effective way to reduce discomfort.

EXPANDED SESSION FRAMEWORKS

Goals: Alleviate pain, calm anxiety, and facilitate emotional or spiritual insight.

1. Opening and Intention Setting (10–15 minutes):

- Begin by inviting the patient to share how they are feeling and what they hope to gain from the session.
- Introduce the session structure, emphasizing the synergy between MHbT, Reiki, and hypnosis.

Sample Practitioner Script: "We'll begin by focusing on your heartbeat to create a sense of calm and connection. As we move into Reiki, you may feel a soothing warmth in areas where you're experiencing pain. Finally, we'll use a guided visualization to help reframe any discomfort you're feeling."

2. Heartbeat Awareness with Reiki (20–30 minutes):

- Perform Reiki hand placements on areas of pain or tension.
- Play an amplified recording of the patient's heartbeat or guide them to feel it directly by placing their hands over their chest or wrist.
- Use verbal cues to help the patient synchronize their breathing with their heartbeat.

Sample Prompt: "With each beat of your heart, imagine waves of relaxation flowing through your body, soothing every area of discomfort."

3. Transition to Hypnosis (30–40 minutes):

- Lead the patient into a hypnotic state using the heartbeat as a focus.
- Introduce a visualization tailored to the patient's needs (e.g., imagining their pain as a block of ice melting with each heartbeat).
- Offer affirmations and suggestions to reinforce the patient's sense of control and ease.

Sample Hypnotic Visualization Script: "As you listen to your heartbeat, imagine it as the steady rhythm of ocean waves. Each wave gently washes away your pain, leaving behind only calm and comfort."

4. Reflection and Integration (15–20 minutes):

- Invite the patient to share their experience and any insights they gained.
- Reinforce the techniques they can use independently, such as focusing on their heartbeat to manage pain or anxiety.

CASE STUDY 1: CHRONIC PAIN RELIEF IN ADVANCED CANCER

Linda, a 70-year-old patient with metastatic breast cancer, experienced constant pain in her spine that limited her mobility and caused frequent anxiety attacks.

- Reiki was used to create warmth and energetic flow in

Linda's lower back while her amplified heartbeat played softly in the background.
- During hypnosis, Linda was guided to visualize her pain as *a cloud of smoke*, dissipating with every exhalation.

Linda reported that her pain felt "lighter and more distant" during the session. Over the following week, she practiced the visualization independently, which helped her manage pain between doses of medication.

CASE STUDY 2: PREOPERATIVE ANXIETY IN LIVER TRANSPLANT CANDIDATE

David, a 59-year-old awaiting a liver transplant, experienced debilitating anxiety about the surgery and postoperative pain.

- Reiki hand placements calmed David's breathing while the practitioner guided him to focus on his heartbeat.
- The hypnosis portion introduced imagery of *a strong, steady lighthouse*, with David's heartbeat as its guiding beacon, representing his strength and resilience.
- David described feeling "calmer and more grounded" after the session. His care team noted reduced anxiety levels during preoperative preparation.

ADVANCED TECHNIQUES AND VISUALIZATIONS

Visualization 1: Pain as a Shifting Sand Dune

- Patients imagine their pain as a *sand dune being reshaped by the wind*, gradually diminishing in size with each heartbeat.
- *Guided Prompt:* "With every beat of your heart, the wind carries away more grains of sand, until only smooth, gentle ground remains."

Visualization 2: Heartbeat as a Flowing Stream

- Pain is visualized as *leaves floating on a stream*, carried away by the heartbeat's rhythm.
- Guided Prompt: "Imagine each leaf as a small piece of discomfort, gently drifting away with the current of your heartbeat."

INTEGRATION WITH PAIN RELIEF DRUGS

Premedication Use: Reduce anxiety before administering opioids, enhancing the patient's receptivity to pain relief.

Post-Medication Use: Sustain comfort and emotional calm after pharmacological interventions.

The integration of *MHbT, Reiki, and Clinical Hypnosis* offers a transformative path to managing *pain and anxiety*, addressing not only the body but also the mind and spirit. As an integrative or stand-alone therapy, this approach empowers patients to reclaim their sense of peace and comfort, creating meaningful relief in life's most challenging moments.

REFLECTION
THE RHYTHM OF HEALING

As we reach the close of this exploration into Meditative Heartbeat Therapy (MHbT) and its integration with Reiki and Clinical Hypnosis, we are reminded of the profound power of connection. This connection is not just to the body, but to our deeper selves, to others, and to the rhythms of life that pulse through all of us. In the steady cadence of the heartbeat, we find not only the physiological rhythm that sustains us, but also a universal pulse that reverberates across emotions, experiences, and our shared existence. It is a rhythm that reminds us we are part of something larger—a movement of energy, life, and healing.

The heartbeat is much more than a biological process; it is a symbol of life's continuity, resilience, and the inherent interconnectedness of all living things. It carries us through moments of joy, sorrow, health, and illness. When life feels uncertain or painful, the heartbeat offers a constant, a reminder of our ongoing presence. In times of suffering or reflection, it provides a simple, grounding force —an invitation to be present with the moment and all that it holds.

The practice of listening to the heartbeat, particularly within the framework of MHbT, invites us to recognize this constant rhythm not only as a bodily function but as a metaphor for life itself. This rhythmic pulse—so familiar and yet often overlooked—is a reminder that each moment, each beat, holds meaning. It represents our connection to ourselves and to the world around us.

In the context of integrative therapies like Reiki and Clinical Hypnosis, MHbT takes on an even deeper significance. These healing modalities—each of which draws on energy, intention, and aware- ness—work in harmony with the heartbeat, offering a pathway toward deeper insight, emotional balance, and comfort. They invite us to attune ourselves to this universal rhythm, not as something to be controlled, but as something to be trusted, felt, and embraced. The true nature of healing, in this sense, is not always about fixing or changing what is broken. Sometimes it is about finding peace within what is, and being present with it in a compassionate and nonjudg- mental way.

The experience of suffering extends far beyond the physical body. Pain and anxiety often intertwine with fear, unresolved emotions, and existential questions about meaning, purpose, and the unknown. In moments of illness or transition, these emotional and spiritual dimensions of suffering can feel as heavy as the physical experience itself. This is where the integration of MHbT, Reiki, and Clinical Hypnosis offers a holistic approach to healing—one that doesn't just address the physical symptoms, but also recognizes the deeper layers of distress that may be present.

Through the practices of MHbT, patients are invited to sit with their heartbeat, to listen not only to its rhythm but to the emotions and thoughts that rise in response. In this space, the heartbeat becomes more than just a physiological sound; it becomes a bridge between the body and the mind, a conduit for healing. The flow of energy through Reiki brings a sense of ease and release, helping to soften the edges of pain and anxiety. Clinical Hypnosis allows the mind to reframe experiences, cultivating acceptance and resilience. Together, these therapies create a sacred space where fear can be released, where the unknown can be met with curiosity, and where the present moment can be embraced with grace.

This process offers not only personal healing for patients but also collective healing for families and caregivers. In the shared experience of these therapies, families can find a space of connection, support, and closure. The rhythm of healing is not an individual journey but a communal one, where every heartbeat reverberates outward, touching those who are near. For practitioners, this integration of practices offers tools to navigate the emotional complexity of caregiving, reminding us that we too are part of the larger rhythm of healing.

The integration of these healing practices calls attention to the importance of partnership in care. Just as the heartbeat synchronizes and harmonizes the various parts of the body, the different aspects of care—physical, emotional, and spiritual—must come together in harmony to support the healing journey. This partnership exists not only between the patient and practitioner, but also between families, caregivers, and healthcare teams. It extends beyond the clinical encounter, creating a larger network of support and understanding that acknowledges the interconnectedness of all.

This partnership is also mirrored in the way that MHbT, Reiki, and Clinical Hypnosis work together. Each modality brings its own unique strengths to the process of healing, and when combined, they create a synergy that is greater than the sum of their parts. The therapies are not just isolated practices; they weave together, responding to the unique needs of each individual and fostering a sense of wholeness that transcends any one aspect of the person.

In a world that often prioritizes efficiency and compartmentalization, this holistic and integrative approach reminds us of the importance of seeing and treating the whole person—body, mind, and spirit. It calls on us to move beyond the limits of traditional, reductionist care models and embrace a more compassionate and comprehensive way of supporting those who are suffering.

As we reflect on the possibilities of these integrative approaches, we are reminded that healing is a deeply personal journey. It is not a destination but a continuous process of becoming—of reconnecting with ourselves, with others, and with the world around us. Whether through the focused awareness of the heartbeat, the nurturing flow of

Reiki energy, or the transformative guidance of Clinical Hypnosis, these therapies offer a gentle invitation to pause and reflect. In doing so, they create space for deeper connection to the inner wisdom we each hold.

For practitioners, this work is a call to recognize the sacredness of our role in guiding others through their most vulnerable moments. It reminds us that we are not merely providers of care, but also participants in the shared experience of healing. This partnership with our patients is one that requires humility, compassion, and presence— qualities that are essential to the work of healing.

For patients, these therapies offer an invitation to explore their inner landscapes with curiosity, courage, and openness. It is a space where they can meet themselves without judgment, a space where the pace of healing is set by the body and the heart. In this way, they are empowered to make peace with their experiences, to embrace the fullness of their emotions, and to find comfort in the rhythms of their own being.

For all of us, regardless of where we stand in the process of healing, these therapies remind us that the journey is not solitary. We are all part of the same great rhythm of life, connected by the pulse of the heart and the breath of the world. The heartbeat carries us forward, reminding us that no matter the challenges we face, we are never alone. There is beauty and healing in our shared rhythms, and in each moment, we have the opportunity to listen, to heal, and to connect.

As we continue this journey—whether as practitioners, patients, or caregivers—we are invited to listen to the rhythm of our own hearts and the hearts of those around us. The heartbeat is a constant companion, guiding us through both calm and storm, joy and sorrow. It offers us a reminder that in each beat, in each breath, we are part of something greater than ourselves—a rhythm of connection, healing, and transformation. Let this rhythm carry us forward, one beat at a time.

CHAPTER II

PALLIATIVE CLINICAL HYPNOSIS AND MHBT

Palliative care, at its core, seeks to relieve suffering and enhance the quality of life for patients with serious or life-limiting illnesses. While conventional medical treatments often focus on alleviating physical symptoms, it is increasingly recognized that truly holistic care addresses not just the body, but the mind and spirit as well. Within this paradigm, complementary therapies such as Clinical Hypnosis and Meditative Heartbeat Therapy (MHbT) have emerged as powerful tools to support both the physical and emotional well-being of patients.

Historically, pain management in palliative care has relied heavily on pharmaceutical interventions, such as opioids, to address physical discomfort. However, these medications often come with significant side effects, including sedation, confusion, and in some cases, dependency Because of these risks,there is a growing interest in non-pharmacological methods that can reduce suffering while avoiding these adverse effects. Clinical Hypnosis has been well-documented as a highly effective means of managing pain, anxiety, and distress, particularly for patients who are nearing the end of life.

When integrated with Meditative Heartbeat Therapy (MHbT), Clinical Hypnosis offers a transformative experience that connects patients to a deep, intrinsic part of themselves—the rhythm of their own heartbeat. This connection to one's internal rhythm is profoundly grounding, offering a sense of security and comfort that can be particularly beneficial for those facing the profound uncertainty of terminal illness.

The integration of hypnosis with MHbT creates a unique, patient-centered approach that provides a rich, multi-dimensional method of healing. MHbT itself is centered around the patient's own heartbeat, an auditory cue that can help to soothe, calm, and center the mind and body. The pulse of one's own heartbeat becomes a form of rhythmic entrainment, facilitating deep relaxation and allowing the patient to enter an altered state of awareness. This deepened state of consciousness allows the individual to explore their physical pain, emotional suffering, and spiritual concerns in a safe and controlled manner, offering a pathway toward healing and acceptance.

The process of Palliative Clinical Hypnosis (PCH) with Meditative Heartbeat Therapy begins with an intention to create a peaceful, safe environment where the patient can fully relax and surrender to the therapeutic process. This journey is designed to unfold through several key phases, each one building upon the last to deepen the patient's connection to themselves, their pain, and their inner sense of peace.

The first phase of PCH with MHbT involves the patient listening to a recording of their own heartbeat. The heartbeat is an ideal anchor because it is profoundly personal—it is the sound of life itself, a constant rhythm that carries the individual through every moment of existence. The sound of one's heartbeat brings the patient back into their body, into the present moment. It can act as a form of grounding, reminding the patient of their ongoing life force.

For many patients, particularly those with advanced illness, the presence of their heartbeat can be a deeply soothing sound. It serves as an auditory confirmation that they are still alive, that there is still time, and that the body is still functioning. This simple act of focusing on one's own heartbeat can foster a sense of security and safety in an otherwise uncertain time.

As the patient listens to the steady beat of their heart, they are guided to relax deeply and settle into a comfortable position. They may lie on their back, sit in a chair, or choose any posture that allows them to feel both comfortable and open to the experience. The clinician's voice helps to guide the patient's focus, leading them into a relaxed state. The focus on the heartbeat draws their attention inward, creating an almost meditative state.

Alongside the sound of the heartbeat, the patient is often guided to focus on a small light, typically a candle flame. The flame serves as an additional focal point, helping to further concentrate the patient's attention and minimize external distractions. The act of focusing on the flame naturally encourages relaxation, as the patient's gaze softens, and the mind slows its constant chatter.

Flame gazing is an ancient technique used in meditation practices across cultures, and it proves especially effective in hypnosis. The flickering flame offers a visual anchor that is soothing to the eyes and mind. Combined with the heartbeat, it creates a dual focus—one auditory, one visual—that helps guide the patient into a deeper state of calm.

The patient is encouraged to synchronize their breath with the rhythm of their heartbeat. As they inhale and exhale in tandem with their heartbeat, they begin to enter a more deeply relaxed state. This process is often referred to as "rhythmic entrainment," where the patient's physiological rhythms align with their breath and heartbeat. This synchronization deepens the trance state, which can further promote a sense of inner peace.

Once the patient has settled into a relaxed position, the therapist gently guides them into the next phase—deepening. This phase of PCH with MHbT allows the patient to release any residual tension in their body. The therapist may use gentle verbal suggestions to encourage the patient to let go of any tightness in the body, allowing each muscle group to relax, one by one, from head to toe.

As the patient becomes more deeply relaxed, they are encouraged to let go of any distracting thoughts or anxieties. This process helps the patient shift from their everyday consciousness into a more fluid, relaxed state, where the body and mind are no longer dominated by stress, pain, or worry. In this state, the patient may experience a profound sense of calm, reducing the impact of physical discomfort and emotional distress.

This deepening phase has been shown to have powerful effects in reducing symptoms such as insomnia, chronic pain, and agitation, all of which are common in palliative care. The hypnotic state allows the patient to temporarily escape the intensity of their suffering and enter a space of peace.

As the patient enters a deeper state of trance, the therapist may introduce the option of guided visualization. In this phase, the patient's subconscious mind is more open and accessible. Visualization techniques can be used to guide patients through emotional or spiritual exploration.

Many patients experience unresolved grief or anxiety as they approach the end of life. In these cases, visualization can offer them a way to process these emotions in a safe, controlled environment. Patients may be encouraged to visualize themselves in calming, healing spaces—perhaps a tranquil garden, a peaceful meadow, or a serene ocean. These imagined environments help to calm the nervous system and bring the patient into a deeper sense of emotional and spiritual peace.

Other forms of visualization can address specific concerns that arise in palliative care. For instance, patients may be guided to visualize meeting deceased loved ones, thereby offering a sense of closure or emotional healing. Alternatively, they may engage in symbolic imagery that is meaningful to their personal or spiritual journey, whether that be through imagery of light, release, or transcendence.

Some patients choose to confront their fears directly, such as the fear of death or the fear of the unknown. In this case, the therapist can guide the patient to visualize themselves embracing these fears, seeing them as a part of the natural cycle of life. This can be an extremely powerful way for patients to release anxiety and come to a place of acceptance, peace, and even transcendence.

In this deeply relaxed state, patients are not only addressing physical pain but also exploring the existential and spiritual dimensions of their illness. Through the integration of both the heartbeat and visualization techniques, the patient is empowered to engage in a holistic healing process that addresses the body, mind, and spirit.

One of the core benefits of Palliative Clinical Hypnosis with Meditative Heartbeat Therapy is its ability to address the multifaceted nature of pain. While physical pain is often the most immediate concern in palliative care, patients also experience emotional and spiritual pain, such as anxiety, fear, and existential distress. This holistic approach—integrating the patient's own heartbeat with hypnosis—creates a therapeutic experience that is not only effective in managing physical pain but also in providing emotional and spiritual relief.

In addition, Clinical Hypnosis has long been recognized as a powerful tool for managing pain. By guiding the patient into a deeply relaxed state, hypnosis can reduce the perception of pain, making it more manageable. In PCH with MHbT, the patient's own heartbeat serves as a grounding anchor that deepens this process. As the patient listens to the familiar rhythm of their heart, it encourages a sense of internal stability and security, allowing them to detach from the intensity of their pain.

Research consistently supports the effectiveness of hypnosis for reducing pain. Studies have demonstrated that hypnosis can lead to significant reductions in pain perception in patients with various forms of chronic or terminal pain. In the context of palliative care, the integration of the patient's heartbeat into the therapeutic process enhances this effect, providing a deeper level of emotional comfort.

Sleep disturbances are common in patients with advanced illness. The anxiety associated with the end of life, coupled with physical discomfort, can make it incredibly difficult for patients to experience restful sleep. PCH with MHbT offers a gentle and natural pathway to restful sleep by leveraging the soothing effect of the heartbeat and the deep relaxation induced by hypnosis.

The rhythmic beat of the heart, combined with deep breathing, can encourage the body and mind to enter a state of relaxation that facilitates sleep. This is particularly important in palliative care, as lack of sleep can exacerbate feelings of stress, anxiety, and pain. By helping patients achieve more restful sleep, PCH with MHbT improves their overall well-being and quality of life, offering them a reprieve from the fatigue of their illness.

As patients near the end of their lives, they may grapple with existential questions related to death, the meaning of life, and what lies beyond. The combination of hypnosis and MHbT creates a unique space where these spiritual concerns can be explored and addressed in a safe, guided way.

Through visualization techniques, patients may be guided to experience profound spiritual moments—whether that involves revisiting meaningful moments from their lives, connecting with loved ones who have passed, or experiencing a sense of peace with their own mortality. These moments of spiritual resolution can help patients face death with a sense of acceptance and peace, reducing fear and anxiety.

CASE STUDY 1: RELIEVING PAIN AND ANXIETY

Margaret, a 72-year-old woman suffering from metastatic breast cancer, had long struggled with severe pain and anxiety that were poorly controlled by medication. During her hospice care, she was introduced to PCH with MHbT. After just a few sessions, she reported a significant reduction in both pain and anxiety. As she listened to the steady rhythm of her heartbeat and focused on a candle flame, Margaret experienced profound relaxation. Over time, her reliance on breakthrough pain medications decreased, and she described a newfound sense of calm, even in the face of her terminal diagnosis.

CASE STUDY 2: OVERCOMING
INSOMNIA IN PALLIATIVE PATIENTS

John, a 68-year-old man with ALS, had experienced chronic insomnia for months, leading to exhaustion and agitation. Traditional sleep aids provided minimal relief, and he often woke feeling groggy and disoriented. The integration of PCH with MHbT into his nighttime routine made a noticeable difference. By focusing on the sound of his heartbeat and the flame gazing technique, John was able to relax deeply and enter a more restful sleep. Over time, his sleep cycles improved, leading to greater daytime energy and overall better quality of life.

CASE STUDY 3: SPIRITUAL INTEGRATION AT END OF LIFE

Maria, an 85-year-old woman with advanced heart failure, had unresolved grief and a deep fear of death. Through PCH with MHbT, she was guided into a relaxed state where she visualized reuniting with her late husband in a peaceful garden. This visualization brought Maria a profound sense of closure and peace. She reported that after these sessions, her fear of death diminished, and she felt ready for the transition. Maria described the experience as "the most peaceful moment I've had in years," marking a pivotal point in her emotional and spiritual journey.

INTEGRATING PCH WITH
MHBT INTO PALLIATIVE PRACTICE

The integration of Palliative Clinical Hypnosis with Meditative Heartbeat Therapy requires careful planning and training. Clinicians, therapists, and chaplains trained in both hypnosis and MHbT must work together to ensure that each patient's unique needs are addressed. Informed consent and patient comfort are paramount, and all therapy sessions must be tailored to the individual's preferences, emotional state, and spiritual beliefs.

This therapeutic approach can be implemented in various palliative care settings, from hospice to home care, providing patients with access to a deeply personalized and compassionate form of treatment. Whether through addressing physical pain, emotional distress, or spiritual concerns, PCH with MHbT offers a holistic healing experience that can profoundly enhance the end-of-life journey.

REFLECTION
THE DOORWAY BETWEEN WORLDS

The heartbeat and the flame—two primal elements, one inward and one outward. The heartbeat, a steady rhythm that echoes the pulse of life itself, and the flame, a flickering symbol of transformation and illumination. Both are powerful forces, each offering a distinct yet harmonious way to access deeper realms of existence. When these two elements are brought together, they create a bridge, a doorway between the known and the unknown, between this world and whatever lies beyond.

To listen to the heartbeat is to become attuned to the very essence of being. It is an invitation to pause, to enter a space of profound awareness, where one is no longer simply living but *feeling* the act of living. In the rhythmic sound of one's own pulse, there is a profound recognition of existence, of the force that sustains us. In this stillness, the body and the mind begin to synchronize, aligning the conscious with the subconscious. This alignment softens the boundaries of ordinary perception, and in that softness, there is a release—a letting go. Here, time becomes less fixed, more fluid. The past, present, and future intertwine, offering a sacred space where healing can begin. It is a moment of integration, where all parts of the self can come into harmony.

This practice of listening to the heartbeat, of tuning into the body's natural rhythm, can be a deeply personal and intimate experience. It asks no more than presence, a simple attention to the now. For some, this alone is enough—a soothing balm for a restless mind and an unsettled body. The steady pulse is both anchor and guide, offering comfort in its unwavering consistency. The gentle focus on the flame—its glow and its dance—adds another layer of connection. It is a reminder that transformation, like fire, is ever-present, ever-moving, ever-changing. The flame, ever on the move, invites us to witness change without fear, to observe its beauty without clinging to it.

Yet, for others, this moment may offer an invitation to venture further—to explore the liminal spaces that exist just beyond the realm of ordinary perception. In these spaces, words fall away, and understanding transcends the linear. Here, we find the possibility of release: the softening of pain, the lessening of fear, and the gentle unfolding of peace. It is within these spaces that a deeper, perhaps even spiritual, healing may occur. Here, the sense of separation begins to dissolve, and there is a profound recognition that we are all part of something greater, a vast web of interconnectedness that transcends the boundaries of the self.

However, not all seek or are ready for this kind of journey. The door to this space is open to those who wish to step through, but it is never a requirement. Some may choose simply to rest in the rhythm of their own heartbeat and the presence of the flame, finding all that is needed in this moment of stillness. Others may wish to move deeper, but whatever path they choose, it is always theirs alone to walk.

As those who support others on this journey, we do not lead, but accompany. The heartbeat belongs to the individual, the flame is a shared symbol of transformation, and the path is unique to each person. We stand as companions, offering no agenda but simply the presence of support, a safe space for exploration. Our role is not to guide the journey but to stand beside them as they walk through the doorway, allowing them to discover what lies beyond, in their own time, in their own way.

This journey is a reminder that healing is not a destination but a process, an unfolding, and that each step, no matter how small or seemingly insignificant, is a movement toward wholeness. In this shared space, we honor both the mystery and the magnificence of the human experience, acknowledging that each individual, with their own heartbeat, is a doorway to a deeper understanding of life, transformation, and peace.

CHAPTER 12

INCORPORATING MHBT INTO END-OF-LIFE DOULA PRACTICE

I n the final hours of life, the presence of a compassionate guide transforms routine care into a sacred vigil. *End-of-life doulas* traditionally provide holistic support through the dying process, but MHbT emphasizes a unique approach: doulas arrive *only* at the vigil, typically the last 72 hours of life, with no prior relationship to the family or patient. They offer no formal bereavement counseling afterwards; their role is strictly to accompany the dying through their final breaths. This concentrated presence requires sensitivity, respect, and deep awareness of the sacred moment. As one hospice teacher notes, sitting vigil is "a sacred invitation and privilege to share presence with a dying person," ensuring that the individual is *not alone until the moment of death*. In MHbT practice, doulas must honor this limited window—an intimate span in which to witness life's closing chapter and "be a witness and companion with a compassionate, kind, and gentle presence."

Traditionally, many doulas plan weeks in advance with families and chart a "vigil plan," but MHbT practitioners often have no such prior contact. Standard training even suggests meeting families early to customize care (lighting candles, arranging music, choosing rituals). By contrast, MHbT doulas are often on call and summoned only when death is imminent. They arrive with the intention of creating a peaceful, sacred space spontaneously at bedside, bearing in mind that *this is the dying person's final performance* and the doula's presence must neither intrude nor distract from the unfolding mystery. Although no two deaths are alike, doulas using MHbT know the vigil often spans one to three days. During this vigil, every heartbeat counts — the very pulse of life ebbs and flows in counterpoint with each breath. The doula's task is to respect that rhythm, accentuating calm and meaning in each passing moment.

By the time of vigil, tangible signs of dying are evident: pulse and breathing irregularities, cooling skin, slowed circulation. But beyond physiology lies the profound *sacredness of the final hours*. In many wisdom traditions, death is a *transition*, not an end. Doulas and loved ones become "guardians of the threshold," accompanying the dying soul with reverence. One Buddhist teacher writes that as death nears, "the living are honored to be in [death's] presence," because *death itself is a sacred transition*. In these hours, the dying person often drifts in and out of consciousness; hearing remains the last sense to fade, so gentle words, silent meditation, or music can be deeply comforting. Every gesture—a soft hand on the brow, a lullaby hummed under breath, the lighting of a single candle—underscores that *this moment is unique and sacred*.

Culturally, many societies have long recognized the power of sound and rhythm at life's end. The *heartbeat* is among the most primal and meaningful of sounds. In fact, *ancient cultures consistently equated the heart with the soul and mind*. Anthropologists note that for millennia, the heart was considered the very seat of thought, emotion, and spirit. As Dr. Henry Marsh observes, "most languages are littered with references to the heart as the seat of the soul and emotion." Biblical and classical texts (even if not directly quoted) echo this notion: the heart symbolizes one's innermost being. Modern science tells us the heart literally beats *around 100,000 times per day*—billions of pulses over a lifetime—but cultures have always sensed that each heartbeat marks the rhythm of existence. Psalm 22:1 ("My God, my God, why have you forsaken me?") and other spiritual writings implicitly recognize the heart as the vessel of ultimate feeling. As one folkloric saying puts it, to lose a heart's beat is to lose life itself.

Global Traditions further illuminate the symbolic resonance of the heartbeat and sound at life's end. For example:

- *Native American (Plains Indian) Drumming:* The powwow drum is literally called "the heartbeat of Mother Earth." As a Sioux drumkeeper explains, *"Our whole culture centers around the drum. The drum brings the heartbeat of our Earth Mother for all to feel and hear. Whether dancing, singing, or just listening, people around the drum can connect with the spirit."* At powwows, dancers experience communal reunion, but at a vigil, a single steady drumbeat can similarly synchronize human pulses to the cosmos. The drum "sets the pace...echoing the heartbeat of the sacred buffalo," linking life and death through song.
- *Potawatomi Ceremonies:* Among the Potawatomi of the Great Lakes, the very word for drum is *déwégen*, from roots meaning *"sound of a heartbeat."* The drum is venerated as *"the heartbeat of the Nation,"* used only in the most sacred ceremonies and life passages. In these rites, participants implicitly hear their ancestors in the drum's pulse, as if each beat were a living pulse of tribal memory.
- *Yoruba and West African Rhythm:* Across West Africa, drumming is regarded as a conduit to the spirit world. The *orisha* Ayan, lord of music and drums, embodies this belief. As one African spirituality blog notes, *"In African culture, the drum is the main instrument for inducing trance. It does this through mimicking the heartbeat. The drum is the heart of the earth."* Ceremony drums replicate life's pulse so powerfully that people enter states of healing and trance. At an end-of-life vigil, such resonance—even if softly

approached—reminds us of the universality of the life-death cycle.

- *European Medieval Practices:* Medieval Europe, too, recognized sound's power at transitions. In ancient cemeteries, drum circles were revived to honor the dead. Sound therapist Ruth Semple describes gatherings where "the steady pulse of our drums will echo the heartbeats of those who came before, creating rhythmic bridges between then and now, between memory and presence." Participants often report feeling more *alive* among the gravestones as the drums pulse, a phenomenon termed "powerful alchemy." In church lore, the ringing of bells— the *death knell*—solemnly announces the passing, marking a final shared sound for a departed soul. These customs, from drums to bells, underscore that sound and rhythm are universal threads woven through death rites.

In *modern spiritual care*, these ancient resonances find new forms. Music therapists like Brian Schreck have pioneered *heartbeat music therapy*: they record a dying patient's heartbeat (using a stethoscope microphone) and integrate it into a custom song. For example, Tim, a hospice patient, asked his music therapist to *"make a recording of [his] heartbeat, and wove music around it."* They even recorded Tim reading a poem to accompany the heartbeat soundtrack. At Tim's funeral, when the heartbeat song played, loved ones gasped—it was as if Tim were speaking to them one last time. His widow recalls that moment: *"When it first started playing at the funeral, people looked at each other, like, 'Is that Tim?' ... It was just amazing."* Such cases show how *preserving the very rhythm of a life* can become a profound gift to survivors. Likewise, at Cincinnati Children's Hospital, a program with Music Therapist Schreck has enabled families to hear their dying child one final time: *"He records heartbeats of critically ill patients and incorporates them into songs to help families cope with the loss of their child."* Though these examples come from music therapy rather than a doula, they illuminate the emotional potency of sound.

In MHbT as practiced by doulas, the concept is similar: using heart sounds or meditative chanting to ground and honor the dying person's spirit.

Meditative Heartbeat Therapy (MHbT) applies these principles in real time at the bedside. In practice, a doula might use a stethoscope or hand on the chest to become attuned to the patient's pulse. They then help the family and patient synchronize breathing or soft humming to that rhythm. Unlike a formal guided exercise, this isn't a scripted meditation, but rather *attentive listening*: noticing each pause between beats, each sigh that follows. Studies of mindfulness and end-of-life care suggest that *presence* itself can reduce suffering. One review found that hospice patients who engaged in mindfulness or meditation reported *less pain, anxiety, and depression, and greater spiritual well-being*. MHbT leverages that insight: by focusing on the here-and-now pulse, it helps the dying person (and those near them) stay present, peaceful, and connected in their final moments. For instance, when anxiety flares, a doula might very gently count each beat with a family member, encouraging them to breathe in time. In this way the relentless forward march of the heart becomes a lullaby, each beat a reminder of enduring life even as life ebbs.

In all these moments, *symbolism is ever present*. Each pulse is a reminder of what has been and what passes—just one beat out of the perhaps *three billion* that have occurred in an average lifetime. Every heartbeat resonates with a lifetime of memories, joys, and sorrows. It is no wonder the heart has come to symbolize love and life universally. The New Statesman notes that when we are anxious or excited, *"we become aware of our heart pounding"*; this visceral link fuels the belief that love, courage, and the soul itself dwell in the chest. As Henry Marsh wrote, the heart has "always had a central role in human imagination and iconography." When a death doula gently speaks of one's heart, they invoke this rich symbolism. They may say, "Your heart is doing such important work now," or simply sit in silence with a warm hand over the chest, honoring the rhythm as holy. In some traditions, religious or otherwise, the last heartbeat is almost like a final breath of sacred ether. Phrases like *"God has numbered all my days"* capture this sense that each beat is counted in some divine ledger.

It is helpful for doulas to recall that many cultures see death not as a dark void but as a transition into another form of being—often accompanied by sound. In *Buddhism*, for example, death is a moment to become fully aware. Tibetan death traditions use chanting and bells to guide consciousness; this practice advises silence and vigil, allowing the dying person's mind to focus inward. In *Hindu* rites, priests chant Sanskrit mantras (like the *Panchakshari* Om Namah Shivaya) to purify the soul, and the final aarti (lamp ceremony) often involves the mantra "Om" resonating as the body is cremated. The Rig Veda speaks of "becoming immortal among the immortals" during the final rite. Similarly, *Native American* death songs and drumming are meant to honor the spirit. The profound silence that often surrounds a natural death can itself be seen as sacred sound—a sort of *beat* that all of creation shares.

Moreover, the *act of vigil* itself is recognized as sacred in many faiths. Christians have long practiced a vigil wake with prayer and sometimes hymns, ensuring a peaceful last night. Jews traditionally recite *Kaddish* (mourner's prayer) through the night and see the community's silent watch as providing comfort. Pagans or Wiccans might circle the bed with chants of release and thanks. As one hospice educator observes, *"Memento mori"*—remembering death—was not meant to terrify medieval people, but to make life more vivid. In the act of vigil, doulas and loved ones consciously enter that "threshold space" where life and death meet. The *heart* is the natural companion in that sacred space—the one organ that speaks of living while signaling death.

CASE STUDIES

MHbT's power can be seen through examples of families who have experienced it (or related heartbeat practices) during the vigil:

Case 1: A Child's Last Gift. In a pediatric hospice program, a child's final wish inspired a creative use of MHbT concepts. Although not a doula, a music therapist facilitated it: the boy's parents brought a small drum into the hospital. As he lay dying, the drummer kept a steady, soft beat, inviting the family to tap along and sing lullabies. His heartbeat was recorded with a sensitive mic and threaded into a simple lullaby melody. The final recording—the beating of his heart overlaid with his mother's humming—became a treasured keepsake. One journalist notes that Cincinnati Children's has a program where *"heartbeat music recording is now a treasured keepsake after [the child's] death,"* helping siblings and parents cope. In MHbT terms, this scenario shows how integrating familial sounds (the drum, the song) with the child's heart rhythm created a "therapeutic vessel of sound" to hold the family's love and grief.

Case 2: Breathing with the Stranger. In another experience, an elderly hospice patient was unconscious and alone except for her anxious daughter. A volunteer doula arrived when the daughter was tearful and confused. The doula gently placed her hand on the patient's chest, feeling the faint, irregular heartbeat. Softly, she encouraged the daughter to breathe with her mother, guiding each inhalation and exhalation in time with the pulse. As minutes passed, the daughter's sobs quieted. The doula hummed a simple chant—a mixture of "Om" and the patient's favorite hymn, barely audible. Without breaking silence, she paid attention to each beat: *ta-dum... ta-dum... ta-dum...* In that rhythm, mother and daughter found a moment of peace. The patient passed away peacefully shortly after, and though this was an informal narrative (not a published case), it reflects how MHbT techniques—synchronization of breath and heartbeat, respectful chant—can ease fear. The daughter later recalled feeling that in those final breaths, *"I felt like I was holding her heart and letting it rest."* Such stories, while personal, mirror research on mindful presence: even silent witnessing and rhythmic breathing can create profound comfort at death.

Case 3: Cultural Resonance. An indigenous woman from a Pueblo community lay dying in the hospital. Her niece, the family's spiritual liaison, explained to the visiting doula that in their tradition, the drum is the voice of ancestors. The patient had a small hand drum on her bed. Recognizing this, the doula asked if she could lightly play the drum in a slow pulse. With permission, the doula tapped a gentle rhythm reminiscent of a heartbeat, soft enough not to disturb but steady enough to enter the space. As the drum resonated against the pillow, elders chanted a simple prayer in the patient's native tongue, and the family gathered. The combination of drumbeat and chant, synchronized with the patient's diminishing pulse, created a bridge between worlds. When the heart finally stilled, there were no abrupt silences; the final drumbeat seamlessly merged into the family's lullaby. This vigil honored both modern hospice care and ancient tradition. In their terms, the drum became "the heartbeat of Mother Earth" surrounding their loved one, affirming that even as she returned to the earth, her spirit was embraced by community and cosmos.

Each case illustrates a common theme: focusing on the heartbeat (literally or figuratively) invites presence, meaning, and continuity. *MHbT practitioners recognize that the final heartbeats of a person— though physiologically faint—carry immense emotional weight.* When those beats are given space and reverence, rather than just being medical data, they become a powerful source of connection and comfort.

Throughout all these experiences, *symbolic continuity* is evident. A person's very first heartbeat is often remembered as the moment life began; MHbT honors that cycle by making their last beats memorable. In mythology and literature, the first and last breaths are threads of a loom; in practice, the doula may say, "With each beat, life flows out and light flows in." By witnessing even a few of those final pulses—arguably "a few heartbeats out of the two billion" someone has lived—doulas participate in a profound passage. As one seeker of meaning might say, *"Each heartbeat is a stanza in the poem of a life."* In these vigil hours, that poem is completing its final lines, and the doula's silent presence is an honored reader.

In conclusion, Meditative Heartbeat Therapy enriches the end-of-life vigil by tapping into deep human and cultural truths about the heart and sound. By aligning mindfulness practice with the living pulse, doulas help families face death not with fear, but with awe and love. This chapter has explored how the simple act of paying attention to the heartbeat—through breathing, chanting, drumming, or recording—transforms clinical care into a *sacred collaboration*. In doing so, MHbT preserves the sanctity of those last precious beats and reminds us all that in the silence after the final heartbeat, love's echo still remains.

REFLECTION
THE SACRED RHYTHM OF LIFE AND DEATH

The integration of Meditative Heartbeat Therapy (MHbT) into the practice of death doulas brings us face-to-face with the profound connection between life and death. The heartbeat is more than just a physical pulse—it is a symbol of the rhythm of life itself. Through the steady beat, we are reminded of the cyclical nature of existence, of the delicate balance between living and dying.

As death doulas, we are called to hold space during this transi tion, to bear witness to the sacredness of each individual's journey. MHbT offers us a way to remain grounded in that sacredness. It provides a rhythm to the process, a gentle reminder that even in the final moments, life continues in a different form. The sound of the heartbeat is a bridge—connecting us to our bodies, our loved ones, and to something greater than ourselves.

When we offer the heartbeat to those we serve—whether it's the dying individual, their family, or ourselves as caregivers—we create a space of peace, connection, and continuity. We offer the dying a steady presence, and in return, we are reminded of the timeless rhythm that flows through all living beings. MHbT, when used with intention and care, allows us to be present in this most sacred of experiences: the passing from life to death.

As we incorporate these techniques into our practice, let us remember that the heartbeats we listen to are not merely sounds. They are sacred rhythms that remind us of the fragile beauty of life and death, guiding us through each moment with reverence, compassion, and grace.

CHAPTER 13

BREATH AND FLAME: INTEGRATING MHBT WITH SUPPLEMENTAL OXYGEN

B y the time supplemental oxygen is introduced in hospice, the body has already begun its long journey toward release. Yet within this medical intervention lies an invitation—a chance to return to the sacredness of breath. This chapter examines the unique integration of MHbT with oxygen therapy, reimagining the flow of air not just as medicine, but as grace.

I kneel by the gentle light of a candle, its flame dancing in tune with the faint hum of the oxygen concentrator standing vigil at the bedside. The night is still, but here everything is alive: flickering orange flame and the slow rise and fall of a human chest in rhythm together. On the white pillow, your head turns slightly as you breathe —patiently, beautifully.

Each inhalation, fueled by the flow of supplemental oxygen, is a little miracle. Each exhalation is a letting go, a farewell to pain and a prayer cast into the night.

In this quiet room, the eternal elements combine: fire and air, breath and heart. The candle flame consumes the very air we breathe, just as breath consumes the air for you and me. One breath feeds the flame; the next breath is fed by it. Here, at the threshold of life and death, these exchanges become a profound metaphor. To breathe here is to enact a sacred dance of elements.

I remember other nights at the bedside. Patients on oxygen depend on that humming machine, and yet in the hush they sometimes find a strange peace. Once I placed a hand on a chest and felt a steady heartbeat amid the whoosh of oxygen flow; the patient's eyes softened. In moments like that, the concentrator's steady hiss becomes part of a quiet symphony—its noisy presence a kind of lullaby. This is the heart of Meditative Heartbeat Therapy: to meet the science of breathing with the soul's stillness.

In medical training we memorize flow rates and oxygen saturations, but seldom do we learn the poetry of a breath. Here, every liter of oxygen can also be a liter of love. Meditative Heartbeat Therapy teaches us to breathe with intention. It invites us to reframe that whirring machine not as an impersonal device, but as a sacred companion on this final journey. In this chapter we weave the ancient symbols of breath and flame with the practical realities of oxygen therapy. We will offer guidance and reflection: an intimate, reverent invitation to breathe love into every moment of care.

Breath has always been sacred to humanity. In many faiths and philosophies, inhalation is synonymous with spirit, life, and the divine. The Hebrew word *ruach*, the Greek *pneuma*, the Sanskrit *prana*, and the Latin *spiritus* all mean both wind and soul. We begin life as dust and spirit, and we return again to the elements of earth and air. In Genesis, God breathes into Adam the breath of life; in the Upanishads, breath is the cosmic fire of creation. In one Native American tradition, a prayer may begin with a deep inhalation to invite the Great Spirit, each breath an offering of thanks.

Even in science, breath has weighty meaning. Every inhale delivers oxygen that our blood carries to nourish every organ, and every exhale returns carbon dioxide to the earth. Bone and muscle depend on this invisible element, and so does consciousness. Without oxygen, the mind becomes clouded, thoughts scatter like smoke, awareness dims. Each exhalation completes a circle: we release carbon dioxide back to earth even as our lungs once drew in what dinosaurs and ancient forests breathed out. The physiology of breath is a quiet miracle of exchange, a reminder that we are intimately connected to all living things — breathing the same air that dinosaurs once exhaled and feeding the forests that feed us.

In poetry and dream, breath speaks in metaphors and mysteries. It is the wind that carries prayer up to heaven, the tide that washes over shore and soul alike, the flame that pulses in a candle and in the human heart. Air is our sweetest necessity, an invisible gift sustaining us, and each breath is an act of communion. To breathe is to commune with the universe: each inhale might be seen as drawing in love, each exhale as a gentle release of all that we must let go. In the sacred chamber of dying, breath itself becomes a teacher. Each gentle exhale is a hymn of release; each grateful inhale, a prayer.

Supplemental oxygen is a staple of hospice care, a therapeutic support for failing lungs and weary hearts. When conditions like advanced COPD, congestive heart failure, or lung cancer cause breath to feel like wading through an invisible deep, oxygen therapy is prescribed to ease the struggle. This is not about prolonging life at all costs, but about bringing comfort and peace. Each liter of oxygen flowing through the mask or cannula is a gift of ease to overworked lungs, a whisper of relief to the body.

Yet this gift comes with a physical presence we cannot ignore. The oxygen concentrator stands at the foot of the bed, humming softly like a mechanical guardian, drawing unseen sustenance from the air. Thick tubes curl over pillows like gentle vines, feeding every breath into the patient's lungs. Portable tanks—heavy with silent promise—rest quietly in a corner, as though filled with bottled angels. The nasal cannula's cool prongs tease at the nostrils, a strange but tender talisman of life. Sometimes a mask is used instead, resting lightly around the face like a soft crown of safety. All of these are part of the patient's world now: a forest of tubing and devices, each strand necessary to sustain the breath.

Dependence on supplemental oxygen often brings ambivalence. Some patients feel tethered or even trapped by the tubes and wires. They may sit quietly tracing the tubes with their fingers or ask anxiously if the machine will quiet when they stop breathing. Others greet it with a childlike awe, grateful for the simple relief when a breath that once burned now comes cool and easy. Clinically, we note practical troubles: nasal cannulas can dry and crack the nostrils; masks can bruise the skin; high flow rates can parch the throat. Nurses offer saline sprays and gentle padding, but the machine still demands daily maintenance—replacing tubing, refilling humidifiers, adjusting settings—while the patient rests.

In the final days, conversations often turn to the role of oxygen. Families wonder, "Is too much oxygen prolonging his life beyond what's natural?" We gently explain that when someone is near death, oxygen can keep organs going, but our focus remains on comfort rather than a stopwatch. Ethically, each person has the right to refuse life-sustaining therapies—including oxygen—if it no longer aligns with their goals. Yet many find that removing oxygen feels like extinguishing a light, even as we reassure them that what matters most is honoring ease and dignity. In these moments, the clinician's task is twofold: to wield medical tools skillfully, and to hold space for questions of meaning.

For us caregivers, the oxygen machine becomes part of the landscape of care. Its hum need not be an intrusion but can become a lullaby of life if we listen with our hearts. In this way, the clinical reality of oxygen therapy—its noise, its tubes, its very presence—can itself be transformed by the reverence we bring to the bedside.

What if we turned toward the oxygen concentrator with gratitude rather than frustration? In many homes, that humming box is nothing less than the breath of life itself. It is a mechanical angel at the foot of the bed, kneeling with us each night. Its steady hum can be heard as a song of mercy. Its long tubes reach out like warm arms, cradling each breath. Even the cool prongs at the nostrils can seem like a gentle halo of air placed by unseen hands. If we imagine the concentrator's machinery as a sacred companion, its very presence becomes a silent gift. Each mechanical breath it gives is mercy incarnate.

Clinically, of course, the machine is just an air pump, but symbolically it is much more. When we adjust the flow or change a tank, we engage in a ritual of care. A caregiver might pause, kneel, and quietly say, "We are adding a little more life to your lungs," transforming a technical duty into a blessing. Each routine task—checking tubes, cleaning a mask, refilling the oxygen reservoir—becomes a ceremony of compassion. The caregiver's hands are both scientific and sacred: in one moment they dial liters of oxygen, in the next they cradle life. There is sacredness in these ordinary actions if they are done with love.

Even the noise of the concentrator can deepen this companionship. That persistent whoosh or buzz becomes a voice of generosity. Instead of an unwelcome clamor, we can hear it saying, "I am here with you." When the machine's pulse clicks in time with the heart monitor, it joins a choir of care. And in those final vigil hours, when silence falls heavy, this symphony of devices underscores the sacred watch. We listen with our hearts to that machine—our fellow breather—and find peace in its constancy.

Just as every breath sustains the body, every breath fans the flame within. Fire has long been a symbol of life and transformation. Consider the candle at our side: as it breathes in air, it brightens, and with every flicker we feel warmth and hope. So too does each inhalation of pure oxygen light our inner spirit. Many traditions speak of an inner fire or light — the spark of life that animates us. As the flame before us requires oxygen to burn steadily, so our heart's flame of hope and presence is fed by every careful breath we draw. In the stillness, the meeting of breath and fire reminds us that life is a dance of give-and-take, of holding on and letting go.

To integrate MHbT with oxygen therapy, we start with gentle observation of breath and heartbeat. A simple practice is to place a hand on the patient's chest or wrist and feel their heartbeat. Together, we breathe slowly, deeply, in a shared rhythm. If the patient is conscious, we might whisper a gentle mantra on each breath: "I inhale compassion; I exhale love," or "I release fear" as the breath goes out and "I embrace peace" as it comes in. The oxygen flowing through each breath can be imagined as *cleansing light filling the lungs*, each exhale releasing tension to the flame.

Even if the patient is no longer responsive, the caregiver's own centered breathing still brings calm. We sit beside the bed, aligning our breath with the machine's hum. Watching a candle flame or a dim light, we breathe in tandem: inhale as the flame grows stronger, exhale as it settles. With each pump of the concentrator, we envision love reaching the patient's heart. When we adjust the oxygen equipment, we do so with reverence: a quiet blessing accompanies each clink of tubing or turn of a dial, turning a routine task into a sacred ritual.

FRAMEWORK FOR PRACTITIONERS: OXYGEN DEPENDENT PATIENTS

1. *Center with Compassion:* Begin each visit by quietly breathing with the patient, aligning your breath with theirs. This shared inhale establishes a bridge; your calm presence can help slow and steady their own breathing. Offer a gentle greeting or touch, acknowledging the patient's effort with each breath.

2. *Listen to the Breath:* Before adjusting any flowmeter, simply observe and honor their breath. Listen to its sound and feel its rhythm. Comment on its beauty or steadiness: "I hear your breath; it's working hard for you." Such validation conveys respect for the patient's life force and reduces anxiety.

3. *Educate with Metaphor:* Explain oxygen therapy in warm, easy terms. For example, liken oxygen to a kind wind helping the lungs. Describe the concentrator as a friend quietly breathing alongside them. Reframe medical details—flow rates, saturations—in the language of comfort ("just enough breeze to fill your sails") to maintain hope and understanding.

4. *Guide Gentle Breathing:* Teach very simple breathing exercises during the visit. You might say, "Let's take one long, slow breath together," then demonstrate a calm inhale and slow exhale. Encourage them to try it, perhaps placing a hand lightly on their chest. Instruct them to imagine inhaling light or warmth. These practices enhance oxygen exchange and instill a sense of inner peace.

5. *Sync Heart and Breath:* If possible, place a stethoscope or hand on the patient's chest or wrist to feel the heartbeat. Encourage them to notice that steady pulse. You can even breathe in rhythm with their pulse for a few cycles. Point out the connection: "Your heart is like a drum giving beat to each breath." This awareness of heartbeat can be deeply soothing.

6. *Harmonize the Environment:* Adjust the setting to be serene. Lower harsh lights, close the door, or light a candle safely nearby if allowed. The glow of a flame or soft music can complement MHbT. Turn off other machines or sounds that are non-essential. Create a cocoon where breath and heart are the focus, not alarms or bright distractions.

7. *Address Physical Comfort:* Ensure oxygen delivery is as comfortable as possible. Check that the cannula isn't too tight and that humidifiers are moistening the air, with the skin protected by soft padding or ointment. A comfortable body helps facilitate relaxation. When repositioning the patient or mask, do so mindfully—explain each step as part of caring ritual and do it slowly with presence.

8. *Encourage Mindful Connection:* Involve family members or caregivers. Invite a loved one to place a hand on the patient's heart or shoulder. Speak softly together, perhaps sharing a few words of gratitude or hope. Teach them the basics of MHbT as you hold the patient's hand through a breathing round. Community presence amplifies the sense of love.

9. *Reflect and Document:* After the visit, note how the patient reacted—did they seem more at ease? Did breathing become more regular? These observations guide future care. Reflect on how integrating MHbT influenced the encounter. Over time, this reflection reminds the team of the spiritual depth in everyday moments of care.

FRAMEWORK FOR END-OF-LIFE DOULAS: LAST 72 HOURS

1. *Prepare a Sacred Space:* Ensure the environment is calm and safe. Dim the lights or light candles, and remove harsh noises. Arrange a gentle fire or flickering lamp if possible. Place meaningful objects or photos near the patient. Position yourself at the bedside so you have direct physical presence. A comfortable chair and your focused attention are essential; the space itself should invite reverence and quiet contemplation.

2. *Center Yourself First:* Take a few slow, deep breaths and ground your presence before engaging with the patient. You are both a witness and a guide now. Clear your mind of other concerns and bless this time with your full attention. If helpful, recite a silent prayer or intention to hold a safe, compassionate space for the dying. Your centered calm can be the anchor in the coming hours.

3. *Mirror the Breath and Heart:* Sit beside the patient and match your breathing to theirs. Lay a hand gently on their chest or wrist, feeling the rise of each breath and beat of each pulse. Breathe as they breathe — in slowly, out slowly — encouraging any lingering effort. This mirroring conveys solidarity and trust. If the patient breathes irregularly, breathe even more softly, exuding calm; your steady rhythm can help anchor the patient's turbulence.

4. *Use Gentle Guided Breathing:* If the patient is receptive, invite one final shared breath. You might softly say, "We

will breathe together." Breathe in with them for a count of
four, hold for two, and exhale for six. As they exhale, you
could whisper a comforting phrase like, "You are safe," or
"Peace surrounds you." These simple practices can quiet
restlessness, easing the transition from struggle to
serenity.

5. *Encourage Symbolic Release:* Help the patient visualize
letting go. For example, guide them to imagine each
exhale as a golden stream carrying away pain and fear. On
the inhale, picture nurturing light filling the body. The
"pulse" of the oxygen flow can symbolize life force. You
might quietly affirm, "With each breath you release what
you no longer need." These symbolic rituals transform
fear into trust and open the heart to surrender.

6. *Attend to Rituals and Customs:* Respect the patient's spiritual
or cultural practices in the final hours. Light incense, play
hymns, or offer a prayer if desired and appropriate. The
oxygen tube itself becomes part of the ritual—when you
change the cannula or mask, do it with gentle reverence,
as if adjusting a crown of air. Invite clergy or loved ones to
join, either silently or aloud, to pronounce blessings or
sacred words as breath quiets.

7. *Support Family Presence:* The family often feels intense
anxiety about each breath. Quietly coach them: "Place a
hand on their chest and take a slow breath together."
Teach them to breathe softly, to whisper words of love
with each exhale. Encourage them to thank each breath,
holding space alongside the patient. Remind them that
their presence and calm breathing convey love beyond
words and that this act of solidarity is a profound gift.

8. *Manage Physical Comfort:* Ensure the patient's body is at
ease. Use pillows to support weary limbs, ease any tension
in the neck, and moisten the lips if dry. If secretions
gurgle, gently turn the head to the side and passively clear
saliva if needed, doing so with prayerful intention. Apply a

cooling cloth to the forehead or a soothing balm on the skin as appropriate. Each small touch or adjustment is a compassionate blessing when given with mindfulness.

9. *Acknowledge Signs of Transition:* As breathing patterns change — Cheyne-Stokes cycles, long pauses, or rattling sounds — gently explain to the family that these are natural steps toward the end. Continue the quiet MHbT practices even as breath becomes sparse. Sometimes no words are needed; your steady presence and the rhythm of a heart-bound prayer can be enough. Offer gentle reassurance, honor the sacredness of the moment, and remain fully present.

10. *Honor the Passing:* When the final breath comes, do not rush. Remain with the patient in reverence. You might hold the hand lightly or stroke the brow. After the breath, simply sit in silent gratitude for a few moments. Softly invite the family to say goodbye in their own way. The flame you lit, the breath you shared, and the heartbeat you held have guided the soul. Allow yourself and the family to reflect, in tender silence, on the sacredness of this journey.

EMBRACING THE BREATH AND FLAME

In weaving breath and flame at life's end, the ordinary becomes utterly sacred. Each moment of oxygen-fueled breathing is recognized as a final prayer, every heartbeat a note in the symphony of love. Through our presence, our prayers, and our care, the technology that surrounds the dying becomes imbued with compassion. With MHbT and mindfulness, we transform clinical routine into sacred ritual. In this light, the last breaths are not ends but gifts — illuminated by inner flame and the remembrance that we all share in the air and warmth of life.

CASE STUDY 1: THE WHITE CHAIR BY THE WINDOW

Miriam had always loved the light. Her daughter told us that in her youth she painted only at dawn, capturing what she called *"God's hour."* Now, at the end of her life, she sat beside the same east-facing window, eyes closed, with the filtered sun softening her gray curls. A humming concentrator rested nearby, its long tube coiled around the legs of the white armchair like a thread of grace. Her breaths were shallow, her chest rising faintly beneath a blanket knit decades earlier.

When I entered the room, the air had already been made sacred —not by my arrival, but by love and intention. Her daughter sat on one side of the chair, her hand on her mother's. I sat on the other. We did not speak at first; we simply breathed.

Miriam's oxygen concentrator, steady and constant, let out a rhythmic pulse—a soft whisper in the sunlit silence. I placed my hand gently on her chest and invited her daughter to mirror me on the opposite side. Together we listened to the machine's breath, then to our own. I whispered, "Let us breathe with her, not for her. Just with her." There was no resistance. Miriam seemed to accept us as fellow travelers in that moment.

I then invited both women to synchronize their breath with the heartbeat. "Feel the beat. Inhale slowly... let it be as long as two beats... now exhale... and again." As we continued, the atmosphere shifted. Time thinned. The air—literal and sacred—grew thick with presence.

Then I began softly repeating a mantra: *"This is your life, this is your breath."* It was from Mary Oliver's *Oxygen,* a line that feels as close to benediction as any I know. The daughter began repeating it too, barely audible.

We remained like that for thirty minutes. When Miriam opened her eyes, she looked at her daughter across the room and said, "Keep painting."

She died quietly two days later in that same chair, with the same oxygen tube gently humming at her side. Her daughter told me afterward, "It was like breathing became prayer."

CASE STUDY 2: THE FARMER'S LAST WINTER

Howard had the strong hands of someone who had turned the earth for decades. His face, weathered by sun and time, was now slack and pale, turned toward the ceiling. He had been unconscious for 14 hours. The room was dim, the air crisp with winter's edge. The oxygen mask over his face hissed like a distant wind.

The nurse said his vitals were declining. She adjusted the oxygen tubing and added a warm blanket. The hum of the concentrator and the rasp of his mask filled the space.

I sat at his bedside, a doula presence in a quiet hour. I began with silence—no words, just breath. Then I placed one hand over his covered chest, palm down, grounding myself in his rhythm. I began to breathe in time with him. His exhalations were soft and fading, yet consistent.

After some minutes, I took out a candle in a glass jar and placed it on the bedside table. I lit it and whispered, *"This is your fire."* The flame shimmered slightly. I imagined the oxygen in the room feeding it gently, just as it was feeding him.

I began the MHbT rhythm aloud: *"Inhale light, exhale rest."* I repeated it quietly, timed with his breath. I visualized his body receiving this oxygen as if the wind itself was brushing his lungs with grace. I added, "With each breath, let the fire within you find peace."

There were no family, no prayers from kin—but the room was not empty. Something older than kinship was present: the breath of earth itself. I placed a hand on his and whispered one last line from Oliver's poem: *"What does this have to do with love, except everything?"*

His breath slowed. Then stopped. The flame flickered once. I stayed long after the last exhale, bearing witness. The nurse returned and said quietly, "That was beautiful."

CASE STUDY 3: A CHILD'S LULLABY

Ellie loved lullabies. She knew she was dying, and her parents had told her with honesty and softness. Her breath was ragged, aided by a small, colorful BiPAP mask decorated with stickers of stars and flowers. When awake, she preferred the nasal cannula, which let her speak and sing.

On her final morning, the nurse—Sarah—offered to guide an MHbT practice with her parents. Ellie agreed. "As long as we get to sing," she whispered, and everyone laughed gently.

Sarah dimmed the lights and lit a small purple LED candle on the nightstand. "Ellie, I'm going to teach you a heartbeat song," she said. "You already know it. You've had it since before you were born."

She gently placed Ellie's hand on her own chest, and her parents followed. "This is the beat of life. Let's all listen."

Together they sang a slow, soft version of "Twinkle Twinkle Little Star," in time with the breath and pulse. Sarah whispered between verses, *"Your breath is starlight, your heart is the night."*

Ellie asked, "Is the machine singing too?"

"Yes," Sarah said. "It's singing with us. It's a very old song."

Ellie smiled. "Okay."

She died that night, peacefully, with her parents on either side, singing. The BiPAP machine hummed softly through the darkness. Later her mother said, "It didn't feel like a machine anymore. It felt like a lullaby keeper."

CASE STUDY 4: THE WHISPER IN THE CATHEDRAL

Eva had lived through two world wars and could still recall the name of her childhood dog. She was mostly nonverbal now, responding only to music and touch. The staff described her as "somewhere between here and there."

On my visit, I brought a small speaker and played Gregorian chant. I sat at her side and rested a hand on her shoulder. The oxygen tube gently looped across her cheek. I began breathing with her—not imposing a rhythm but simply joining hers. The hum of the oxygen concentrator blended with the voices of the chant.

After a few minutes, I quietly repeated a phrase: *"Peace to your breath, peace to your flame."* I then placed a small, wooden heart-shaped token on her nightstand. Her great-niece joined us, eyes closed, silently placing a hand on Eva's hand. We sat that way for nearly 40 minutes. No one spoke. The only sounds were the chant, the concentrator, and the shared breath of love.

When Eva passed later that week, the great-niece emailed me: "She always loved cathedrals. I think you turned her room into one."

ETHICAL AND EXISTENTIAL DIMENSIONS OF OXYGEN AT THE END OF LIFE

There are few interventions in hospice care as symbolically potent—and as emotionally loaded—as supplemental oxygen. It is the quiet bridge between presence and absence, struggle and surrender. It does not cure, and in most cases near the end of life, it no longer prolongs. Yet the oxygen tube, the mask, the ever-humming concentrator, often becomes the last thread binding a person to this world. It is the breath made visible. The fire sustained by invisible wind.

To touch the oxygen dial is to touch something sacred.

In hospice care, the question is not *whether* someone will die, but *how*. When a patient becomes oxygen-dependent, the intention behind its use must be clarified and revisited gently.

Oxygen therapy is often introduced with the goal of easing breathlessness. But for some patients and families, oxygen may be seen—consciously or not—as a means of "keeping them alive." This creates a quiet ethical tension.

A daughter might say, "Don't turn it off, I don't want her to die." A nurse might think, "She's not really benefiting anymore." A patient might plead, "It helps me feel like I'm still here."

The role of MHbT in these moments is not to argue for or against oxygen, but to hold the conversation with sacred attentiveness. The breath is not only physiological—it is theological. It carries memory, identity, soul. When we adjust oxygen flow, we are not just opening a valve—we are crossing into the realm of symbol.

- *Intention is key.* If oxygen is being used to relieve suffering, it aligns with hospice ethics.
- *Informed reflection.* Families should be lovingly guided to understand the *why* behind continuing or stopping oxygen.
- *Agency matters.* Patients who are able should be involved in decisions about oxygen use, and their spiritual relationship with breath honored.
- *Avoid binary thinking.* Oxygen need not be "on or off." Sometimes it may be reduced gradually or used only for comfort, not saturation targets.

One of the most compassionate acts a practitioner can perform is to reframe the oxygen not as "keeping them alive" but as *blessing the breath*—making each remaining moment easier, clearer, more peaceful.

There comes a moment in many deaths when the family asks, *"Should we turn it off?"* It may be after the last conscious moment, when breaths are spaced minutes apart, when the mouth opens but does not pull in air, when the body has already begun its luminous withdrawal. The oxygen continues, but the breath is no longer asking for it.

There is no universal right answer. In some traditions, oxygen remains until the very last heartbeat, like incense trailing behind a departing soul. In others, it is gently removed as part of a conscious letting go. Medically, it is rarely required. Spiritually, it may be essential.

What matters most is intention and presence. If oxygen is removed, it should be done with reverence.

A POSSIBLE RITUAL FOR WITHDRAWAL

- Dim the lights.
- Let the family gather.
- Explain softly: *"The oxygen has helped ease the breath. Now that the breath is nearly finished, we can let the machine rest too."*
- Place a hand over the heart as the dial is turned.
- Whisper: *"As your breath returns to the stars, may your heart be at peace."*
- Light a symbolic flame—candle or otherwise—and keep it near.

MHbT can be practiced before, during, and after this moment. The heart continues to beat for minutes after the last breath. In this sacred interval, the practitioner can breathe softly, mirroring what remains, keeping vigil until silence settles fully into the room.

To lose one's breath is not just to die—it is to unravel one's self. Breath is *I am*. It is how we cry, sing, pray, whisper, call for help. For patients facing death, the slowing or labored breath can feel like erosion of identity. "I'm not myself anymore," they may say. "I can't catch my breath." The statement is not only physical—it is metaphysical.

MHbT meets this fear not with solutions, but with presence.

By anchoring the person in their heartbeat, in the hum of the oxygen, in the gentle ritual of sacred attention, MHbT affirms: *You are still here. You are still loved. This is still you.* Even when words are gone. Even when the breath falters.

THE FAMILY'S DILEMMA

For many families, the oxygen machine becomes a line between hope and despair. They listen to it constantly. They fear it stopping. They fear it continuing.

MHbT invites them to shift their relationship. Instead of fearing the concentrator's noise, we invite them to hear it as a blessing. "This hum is the voice of love. It is here with you, not against you." We might sit with them and breathe together, hand on the tube, as if the machine itself were a companion.

When the time comes to consider turning it off, we give them language:

- *"It has done its work."*
- *"The breath is ready to return to the wind."*
- *"You can keep the oxygen going for as long as it comforts you—or let it rest."*
- *"There is no wrong choice here. Love is in both."*

MHbT teaches us to hold ambiguity with grace. Not to resolve the unresolvable, but to bring beauty to the tension.

There is sometimes one last breath. A long pause. Then stillness.

We do not know where the soul goes in that moment, but we know it passes through the door of breath. The oxygen machine may still be humming softly, unaware of the crossing.

That is why MHbT practitioners sit in silence afterward. We hold the breath beyond breath. We continue to listen with our hearts for a few moments more. And then, perhaps, we whisper: *"You have returned to the fire."*

AN IMPORTANT NOTE

There are moments—especially in overnight shifts, rural homes, or under-staffed facilities—when you may be the only one present. No team, no family. Just you, a patient on oxygen, and the quiet hum of night.

In these moments, MHbT becomes something more than technique. It becomes a compact between breath and flame, presence and surrender. You are the circle. You are the firekeeper.

You place your hand on the patient's chest, hear the oxygen pulse, and begin to breathe. You listen not just for clinical changes, but for the subtle music of their soul. You might speak a quiet mantra, or remain in complete silence. You sit as their last companion, bearing witness not only to their death, but to their life.

These moments will change you. You will not be able to speak of them to everyone. But the patient will know.

AT THE HEART of this work—of every moment spent listening to a patient breathe, of every hand placed reverently over a failing heart, of every hum that rises from a concentrator in the corner of a dimly lit room—is a simple truth: *we are made of breath and flame.* And it is breath, not words, that becomes the last expression of a life.

MHbT offers us a spiritual cartography for this journey. It maps no theology and makes no doctrine. It simply teaches us to notice what is already there: the pulse, the breath, the quiet hum of being. And in noticing, we remember: the heart's rhythm is not only a medical metric—it is the memory of dancing, crying, laughing, loving. It is the soul's drumbeat. The oxygen machine, far from an intrusion, becomes a choir member in the final chorus. Its rhythm steadies the room, filling the silence not with noise, but with promise.

At the bedside, we do not need to solve anything. The machine hums. The breath moves. The heart slows. The flame flickers. Our task is to witness—attuned, open, reverent.

Let this chapter close where it began: with a breath.

Let it remind us that to offer oxygen is not merely to deliver air— it is to say, *"Your life still matters."*

To touch the pulse is not merely to measure—it is to say, *"I am with you in this rhythm."*

To sit through the last inhalation is not merely to observe—it is to love.

And in the stillness that follows, when the machine is finally silent and the air no longer moves, may we know that we were part of something sacred. We breathed with them. We kept the flame.

REFLECTION
THIS MERCIFUL MACHINE

There is a moment—sometimes minutes, sometimes hours before death—when the breath slows, and the room feels impossibly wide. The family has stopped speaking. The nurse has made their notes. The concentrator hums steadily, its own breath filling the silence. The patient lies still, but not absent. Something is happening. Not an end, exactly, but a thinning. A quiet surrender. A flicker. And in that moment, I have often found myself holding mine—my breath, that is—as if to make room for theirs.

This reflection is for that moment.

It is not a medical text, though medicine threads through it. It is not a theology, though spirit moves in every line. It is not a eulogy, though it carries the scent of many rooms in which lives have ended. It is a reflection—a long, slow exhale of everything Meditative Heartbeat Therapy has taught me about the meaning of breath at the end of life.

We live our lives on the breath. More than 23,000 times a day, we inhale the world and offer it back again. Most of us never notice. But in hospice rooms—when machines echo the sound of breathing, when oxygen is both the comfort and the tether, when each breath is counted not by lungs but by love—we begin to see: breath is sacred.

Mary Oliver once wrote about sitting beside a loved one on oxygen and realizing that the machine, loud and foreign as it was, had become merciful. The noise itself was a gift. It kept the breath going. It kept love possible. It offered, quite literally, time.

In my own work, I have often asked families to listen. "Just listen to the sound of the oxygen," I'll say. "It's singing with them." Most don't hear it at first. They hear a buzzing, a mechanical drone, an unwelcome reminder of illness. But slowly, something changes. They begin to hear rhythm. They begin to hear life.

And then, eventually, they hear love.

The machine, in all its clinical functionality, becomes a companion. A witness. A final choir member singing under the breath of a dying person. Its whir is not unlike a lullaby—the same hush we might have heard as children falling asleep. That's what makes it so powerful. It returns us to our beginning even as we prepare for our ending.

Breath is circular. And in that circle, MHbT finds its home.

There is a story told by some Indigenous elders of the Northeast: when a person is born, they are given a candle deep within their chest. This candle is not lit until their first breath. The flame is invisible, yet it burns. Through laughter, we feed it. Through sorrow, we shelter it. Through love, we keep it burning bright. And when the last breath leaves the body, the flame flickers outward—not extinguished, but returned to the Great Fire, the Source.

I think of this often as I sit with the dying.

In rooms filled with machines, monitors, tubing, and the ever-present hiss of oxygen, there remains this quiet fire. I have seen it in the eyes of a patient who, despite her pain, turned her head to look at her son one last time. I have seen it in the sudden exhale of someone who had not spoken in days but used their final breath to say, simply, "Thank you." I have seen it in the rise and fall of the chest, even when everything else had failed.

That is what breath is. It is the visible signature of the invisible fire.

And the oxygen we deliver—the machine we position beside the bed, the tubing we loop behind the ears, the mask we gently place—is not just medical equipment. It is kindling.

Too often, we fail to see the sacred in what is ordinary. We forget that the oxygen we prescribe came from the stars. That it was trapped in stone and water, released into the trees, and offered now through human-made machines to someone whose body still wants to stay. This air we give is not just air—it is memory. It has moved through forests, lungs, forests again. It is shared breath.

We are, in a very literal way, breathing one another.

So when we offer oxygen to the dying, we are offering a chance for that person's flame to stay a little longer. Not because we are afraid of the dark—but because the flame still has more light to give.

MHbT teaches us not just to observe the breath, but to become it. To sit in rhythm. To listen for the heartbeat not just with stethoscopes but with presence. When the breath is labored, we breathe slower ourselves. When the breath pauses, we do not panic—we accompany. When the oxygen machine hums in the background, we do not silence it—we bless it.

Because this, too, is holy.

It often begins as resistance.

When patients first encounter the oxygen concentrator, they may flinch at the sound. They ask, *"Does it have to be so loud?"* Or they ask, *"How long will I need this?"* As if the machine's arrival is a herald of finality. As if the soft whir of its breath is too intimate a thing to accept.

I have heard family members call it "that machine," with a tone that falls somewhere between grief and resentment. It is understandable. Its arrival marks a turning point: the body can no longer do it alone. Something has changed. Something cannot be reversed.

But over time, a strange thing happens.

What was once foreign becomes familiar. The noise becomes background music. The tubing becomes part of the bed. The patient begins to reach instinctively for the cannula in the night, like one might reach for the hand of a loved one in the dark. And for many, the oxygen machine becomes a companion. A quiet ally.

A steady friend who asks nothing, gives everything, and simply stays.

I once cared for a man named Joseph who told me that the hum of his concentrator reminded him of the old freight trains outside his childhood bedroom. "I used to fall asleep to that sound," he said, "and now I guess I'll die to it too." He smiled when he said this. Not with despair, but with a kind of peace. "Same sound, different track."

That's when I realized: it's not just oxygen we're delivering. It's continuity. It's meaning. It's the sound of something that stays.

MHbT offers us the lens to perceive this machine differently. Not as invasive, but as intimate. Not as a barrier to sacredness, but as a bearer of it. We can invite patients and families to hear the machine's rhythm as a surrogate heartbeat—something that breathes alongside the one who is dying. Not replacing them, but supporting. Not commanding, but accompanying.

We can say: *"This sound means you are being held."*

We can say: *"This machine is here because your breath matters."*

We can say: *"Let's breathe with it together."*

And just like that, the clinical becomes communal. The machine becomes something else entirely.

Mary Oliver called it merciful. She saw beyond its plastic casing and motorized fan and heard instead the echo of love—pressed through a mask, passed through a prayer, carried into a quiet room by the sacred hush of air.

Oxygen is not only what we give—it is how we stay.

We rarely talk about the soundscape of dying.

We speak of symptoms, comfort, medications. We document respiration rates and oxygen saturation. We chart the pauses between breaths with clinical precision. But we forget that for the dying—and for those who sit vigil beside them—the *sound* of the moment is what remains.

The hush of a room where everyone is holding their breath.

The whisper of a hand stroking a forehead.

The soft tremble of a voice reading Psalm 23 or humming an old lullaby.

And always—if oxygen is flowing—the steady sound of the concentrator.

It is not music, exactly. It is not silence either. It is a sound that lives between worlds: mechanical, yes, but also profoundly alive. It is the sound of something working faithfully in the background of everything else. And if we are quiet—truly quiet—it begins to sing.

Each soft inhale it offers becomes a part of a deeper liturgy. Each push of air through tubing becomes a chant. In the sacred hush of a final night, that sound carries a kind of weight. It says, *This body is still breathing. This soul is still here.*

For those who remain, it becomes a tether. Something to listen to in the dark. Something to mark time by when all other clocks have stopped.

I recall a woman, Anita, whose mother lay dying in a small hospice room. The only light was from the hallway, and the only sound was the oxygen machine. Anita had grown used to it—so much so that she no longer noticed it. But after her mother took her final breath, a nurse gently leaned over and turned the machine off.

The room fell into absolute silence.

And Anita began to weep.

Later, she said to me, "I didn't realize how much I was listening to that sound. It was like she was still here. And when it stopped, I knew she was really gone."

It's easy to dismiss that moment as grief, or as a sentimental attachment to noise. But it was more than that. The oxygen concentrator had become her mother's final music. A breath choir. A heart drum. When it stopped, so did the illusion of time. So did the illusion of breath.

MHbT honors that sound. It teaches us not to fight it, not to mute it, not to apologize for it—but to fold it into the ritual. To let it become the sound that carries someone home. That sound is not foreign—it is familiar. It is a gentle freight train, a night tide, a remembered whisper.

It is a lullaby for the soul.

There is a moment—a strange, suspended moment—when the

person before you is still breathing, but the breath is no longer *theirs*. You can see it. The body inhales, exhales, but the soul has already begun to rise like mist before dawn. The chest moves, but the spirit has grown still.

These are the moments when oxygen becomes ghostlight.

You sit beside them, your hand on theirs, and you can feel the warmth still in the fingers. The machine continues its hum, pumping breath into lungs that no longer reach toward it. It is mercy now by muscle memory alone. A few breaths remain—not to sustain, but to accompany. And here, in this fragile veil between presence and departure, MHbT becomes the tenderest of companions.

You do not guide the breath anymore—you witness it.

You do not speak—you echo.

You do not lead—you listen.

I have sat in such silence many times. Not waiting. Not willing. Just being.

Just breathing.

There is no script for this. No protocol. What you do with your breath becomes the liturgy. What you do with your eyes, your hands, your heartbeat—these are the final offerings.

And still, the machine goes on.

Some families ask, *"Should we turn it off?"* Others whisper, *"Leave it."*

There is no right answer.

But there is this: each breath that continues is no longer a gasp for survival. It is a candle in a window. It is the parting breath of a story told slowly, lovingly, all the way to the final punctuation. The oxygen is no longer giving life—it is giving the *space* in which to let go.

In that space, MHbT becomes silence itself. You breathe, not to guide, but to remember. You place a hand on their chest, not to steady them, but to bless the rhythm that was. You close your eyes and listen to the heartbeat—not with ears, but with the soul.

And when it stops, when the breath no longer stirs the chest, when the flame wavers and finally folds into its source—then and only then, you reach toward the dial.

And with reverence, you turn the machine off.

And the silence that follows is not emptiness.

It is arrival.

I believe we do not die into absence.

We die into return.

Just as oxygen feeds flame, and flame gives light, and light disappears only into light again—so does the soul return to its origin. We are not extinguished. We are released.

I have come to think of death as the moment when the small, private fire within us is drawn back into the Great Fire. Not burned, not erased—but welcomed home. In this way, our final breath is not an ending—it is a spark returning to its source. It is the breath becoming wind. The flame becoming sky.

This is not metaphor alone. I have *felt* it.

I have sat at the bedside of a woman who opened her eyes a final time and whispered, "I'm going back."

I have watched a man reach upward with both hands, fingers opening like embers scattered into the night.

I have seen the moment when the body relaxed—not in death, but in arrival. Something opened. Something lifted.

In MHbT, we do not try to describe that place. We do not claim to chart the terrain of the after. But we do hold vigil at its border. We sit close to the fire. We feel its warmth. And we bless the breath that crosses over.

The oxygen machine hums, and we hum with it. The heart slows, and we match it. The light dims, and we become the lantern.

And then—the fire goes.

Not gone. Not lost.

Just returned.

The oxygen, the heartbeat, the fire within us—none of them are separate.

They are love made audible. Love made visible.

And when the body can no longer hold them, love returns to where it came from. It doesn't end. It disperses.

It becomes the breath of others. The light in someone else's night. The warmth at the center of a candle long after it's been blown out.

The Great Fire does not consume.

It welcomes.

A BENEDICTION FOR THE BREATH

May the breath you give be the breath you receive.
May each inhale you offer in love return to you multiplied—
through silence, through song, through the soft hum of a machine
that knows how to pray.
May you never fear the sound of oxygen.
May it become to you what it became to me:
a kind of lullaby,
a second heartbeat,
a voice that says, *"I'm still here."*
May you hold the hand of the dying with reverence,
not to keep them here,
but to remind them that here was worth being.
May you feel the heartbeat slow, not with dread,
but with awe.
You are witnessing the world exhale something holy.
May you light a candle not in mourning,
but in continuation.
Let that flame remind you: they are not gone.
Only returned.
May you learn to breathe alongside grief—
not over it,
not beneath it,
but with it.
And when the room is quiet,
and the machine has been turned off,
and the last breath has settled into the walls—
May you still hear something.

The memory of rhythm.
The echo of a whisper.
The soul's final sigh.
And may you know, deep in your bones,
that it was never just oxygen,
never just noise,
never just care.
It was love.
It was always love.

CHAPTER 14

OTHER PRACTICAL
APPLICATIONS OF MHBT

USING MHBT TO MANAGE ANXIETY AND STRESS

Anxiety is a prevalent emotional response among individuals receiving palliative or hospice care. The uncertainty surrounding death often triggers heightened emotional responses, including fear, panic, and existential dread. Patients may struggle with anticipatory grief, fear of abandonment, or unresolved conflicts, leading to emotional distress that complicates their physical symptoms.

The psychological impact of terminal illness can manifest in various forms, including:

- *Generalized Anxiety*: Constant worry about the future, treatment options, and the dying process.
- *Panic Attacks*: Sudden episodes of intense fear accompanied by physical symptoms such as rapid heartbeat, shortness of breath, and sweating.
- *Existential Anxiety*: Concerns related to meaning, purpose, and the legacy one leaves behind.

Meditative Heartbeat Therapy offers a structured way for patients to regulate their anxiety by shifting their focus to the steady rhythm of their heartbeat. The practice activates the parasympathetic nervous system, slowing the heart rate and calming the mind.

During MHbT sessions, practitioners guide patients through several steps designed to alleviate anxiety:

1. *Breathing Techniques*: Patients are encouraged to engage in slow, deep breathing to facilitate relaxation.
2. *Heartbeat Listening*: Patients listen to their recorded heartbeat, focusing on the rhythmic sound as a grounding exercise.
3. *Mindful Reflection*: Practitioners prompt patients to observe any emotions that arise during the session, promoting awareness and acceptance.

CASE EXAMPLE: MANAGING END-OF-LIFE ANXIETY

Patient Background: Alan, a 72-year-old man diagnosed with advanced pancreatic cancer, entered hospice care after discontinuing curative treatments. Alan experienced frequent panic attacks, particularly at night, when thoughts of his impending death became overwhelming. His caregivers found it challenging to comfort him, as his anxiety often escalated despite medication.

The hospice team introduced MHbT as part of Alan's care plan. His heartbeat was recorded using a digital stethoscope and played back to him during meditation sessions. Alan described the sound of his heartbeat as "strangely reassuring," remarking that it gave him something tangible to hold onto during moments of fear.

Over time, Alan began practicing heartbeat meditation independently, using the recordings before bedtime to ease his anxiety. The calming effect of the therapy reduced his reliance on sedatives, allowing him to engage more fully in conversations with his family and reflect on his life. Alan's panic attacks decreased in frequency and intensity. He described the experience as transformative: "My heartbeat became my anchor—a way to remind myself that I'm still here, still breathing."

FAMILY-CENTERED MHBT: STRENGTHENING EMOTIONAL BONDS

Family involvement is a critical aspect of palliative care, as patients and their loved ones often need to navigate complex emotions together. MHbT offers a unique opportunity for families to connect emotionally, creating moments of shared presence and intimacy.

The emotional landscape in palliative care can be complex, with family members often grappling with their feelings of grief, fear, and helplessness. Collaborative MHbT sessions provide a platform for families to support one another, reinforcing emotional bonds during difficult times.

Joint MHbT sessions typically involve family members listening to the patient's heartbeat through headphones or placing their hands over the patient's chest. These shared experiences foster empathy and mutual understanding, creating a space for meaningful communication. Practical implementation includes:

1. *Grounding Techniques*: Begin family sessions with grounding exercises to help everyone feel centered and connected.
2. *Heartbeat Meditation*: Utilize the recording of the patient's heartbeat as a focal point for reflection.
3. *Facilitated Discussion*: Encourage family members to share their thoughts and feelings about the experience, promoting open communication.

CASE EXAMPLE: RECONNECTING THROUGH MHBT

Maria, an 84-year-old woman with end-stage heart disease, had become emotionally distant from her daughter, Elena, due to past conflicts. As Maria's condition deteriorated, Elena expressed regret over their strained relationship but found it difficult to engage in meaningful conversations.

The hospice team facilitated a joint MHbT session, where Maria's heartbeat was recorded and played back for both mother and daughter. Elena described the experience as "profound," noting that it gave her a new way to connect with her mother without needing to find the right words.

After several MHbT sessions, Maria and Elena began talking more openly about their feelings. Elena reflected, "Listening to my mom's heartbeat was like hearing the rhythm of our relationship— imperfect, but still beating." This process allowed them to reconcile before Maria's passing, leaving Elena with a sense of emotional closure.

This chapter has presented a series of practical applications of Meditative Heartbeat Therapy (MHbT), emphasizing its role in managing anxiety, strengthening family connections, and fostering community support. MHbT provides patients and caregivers with valuable tools to navigate the emotional complexities of end-of-life care.

The integration of MHbT into holistic care models can significantly enhance the quality of life for individuals facing terminal illnesses. As practitioners continue to explore innovative approaches to care, MHbT stands out as a powerful method for promoting emotional well-being and connection.

REFLECTION
THE RHYTHM THAT CONNECTS US ALL

I n our busy lives, the heartbeat often goes unnoticed, a quiet pulse that sustains us yet fades into the background of our daily consciousness. But there are moments when we pause and listen, when the rhythmic sound of our heartbeat offers a reminder of the simple but profound fact of being alive. This rhythmic pulse, shared by all living beings, is an invitation to find sanctuary within ourselves, even in the midst of uncertainty and fear.

At the end of life, or during times of deep distress, anxiety can feel like a powerful current, dragging us away from the peace that feels so distant. It often brings with it overwhelming questions, fears of the unknown, and an endless swirl of "what ifs." In those moments, the heartbeat offers an unexpected sanctuary. It does not remove the anxiety but creates space for calm within it. By simply bringing attention to the steady pulse within, we are reminded that we are still here, still breathing, still capable of presence—even when everything else seems uncertain. Each beat becomes an anchor, a gentle reassurance that in this moment, we are enough. This is not an invitation to erase fear, but to coexist with it, to find peace amidst it.

The heartbeat, when observed with intention, offers more than a momentary calm—it teaches us the practice of returning to the present. When life feels overwhelming, when the mind races and the future seems unclear, the heartbeat becomes a rhythm that transcends urgency. It reminds us that the pace of life does not have to be dictated by constant doing, but can be found in simply being. In these small moments of stillness, we reconnect to something deeper, a rhythm that transcends the individual self and connects us to the web of all life.

One of the beautiful aspects of the Meditative Heartbeat Therapy (MHbT) practice is its ability to create connection through silence. The simple act of listening to another's heartbeat creates an unspoken bond, a shared experience that transcends language. In a family-centered session, the act of placing a hand over a loved one's chest to listen becomes a profound expression of presence. In that shared silence, words fall away, and the heart becomes a language of its own—a language that expresses love, acceptance, and the unspoken connections that tie us together.

This practice fosters emotional intimacy, offering a way for families to reconnect in moments when words might fail. It provides an opportunity for reconciliation, for the healing of old wounds, for saying what has long been left unsaid. Each heartbeat is a silent message: "I see you. I hear you. I am here with you." There is something deeply human in the rhythm of the heart; it is a reminder of the ways we are all interconnected, of how much can be shared in presence without the need for explanations or fixes.

For those facing the end of life, MHbT offers not just a therapeutic tool, but a way to honor their legacy, not through material accomplishments, but through the way they have shown up for others in love and presence. Families often speak of the profound comfort in listening to a loved one's heartbeat after they have passed, finding solace in the memory of their shared connection. In the steady pulse of the heart, they discover a rhythm that continues to echo beyond the final breath, a living testament to the ways in which we remain woven together even after physical separation.

In the role of caregiver, there is often an unspoken expectation to "fix" things—whether that is alleviating physical pain or comforting emotional distress. MHbT invites us to reconsider this need to "fix." It teaches that the most valuable gift we can offer is not a solution, but our presence. Listening to another's heartbeat is an act of profound stillness. It says: "I am here with you, just as you are." In this presence, the patient is not alone with their fear or pain. They are witnessed, accepted, and affirmed simply through the act of being.

This principle extends far beyond the caregiving relationship. It speaks to the broader human experience—how often do we feel the need to "fix" those we care about, to offer solutions when sometimes what is needed most is our listening ear and undivided attention? MHbT reminds us that presence, not perfection, is what truly heals. By embracing the act of listening without the need to intervene, we create a space where healing can unfold naturally.

There is a quiet lesson embedded in the rhythmic pulse of the heart: our legacy is not measured in what we accumulate, but in the way we show up for others. MHbT encourages us to reflect on the heartbeat not as a symbol of life's end, but as a living embodiment of the way we have lived—of how we have loved, of how we have been present for others, and of how we have chosen to walk through the world.

In listening to the heartbeat, we are reminded that our impact endures long after we are gone—not in material possessions, but in the relationships we have nurtured, the love we have shared, and the moments we have been fully present. The heartbeat becomes a lasting legacy, continuing to echo in the lives of those we leave behind.

One of the most profound aspects of MHbT is its ability to create simple, intentional rituals of connection. These are not grand or elaborate ceremonies, but moments of shared presence. A family gathered around a loved one, placing a hand on their chest to listen to the heartbeat. A caregiver holding space for a patient in stillness. A group of people joining together to listen, to breathe, to share in the rhythm of life.

These rituals hold deep meaning, offering a way to mark significant moments—whether they are moments of transition, of reconciliation, or of gratitude. In a world that often rushes through change, MHbT offers a powerful invitation to slow down, to pause, and to be fully present. It teaches us that connection is not something that happens to us—it is something we create, moment by moment, beat by beat.

As we continue to engage with the practice of MHbT, let us carry the rhythms we have encountered. Let us remember that healing is not something we achieve, but something we cultivate—through presence, connection, and shared experience.

In this rhythm, there is a deep reminder: we are part of something larger than ourselves. Our heartbeat is connected to the rhythms of all those we love, those who have come before us, and those who will come after.

Let this rhythm guide us—not just in times of crisis, but in the ordinary moments of life. Let it remind us to listen deeply, to be present, and to create space for connection. In each heartbeat, we find the rhythm that carries us forward, one beat at a time.

CONCLUSION
AND REFLECTIONS ON
THE JOURNEY OF MHBT

As we reflect on the journey of Meditative Heartbeat Therapy (MHbT), it becomes evident that this innovative approach has the potential to transform the landscape of hospice and palliative care. By centering the therapeutic experience around the patient's heartbeat, MHbT offers a unique pathway for emotional regulation, spiritual connection, and interpersonal bonding.

At the core of MHbT lies the concept of heartbeat awareness, which serves as both an anchor and a guide for individuals navigating complex emotional landscapes. By focusing on their heartbeat, patients can cultivate a sense of presence and connection, allowing them to confront difficult emotions with greater compassion.

The process of tuning into one's heartbeat fosters a sense of safety. Patients report feeling more grounded and connected to their bodies. This connection is vital, especially for those facing terminal illness, where the fear of loss often manifests as anxiety and despair. Heartbeat awareness offers a mechanism for patients to process these feelings constructively, promoting emotional healing.

Throughout the case studies presented, it is evident that MHbT enhances emotional regulation and resilience among patients and families. By engaging in heartbeat meditation, individuals learn to observe their emotions without judgment, fostering acceptance and reducing anxiety. This newfound resilience empowers patients to face the challenges of illness and loss with a greater sense of agency.

CASE EXAMPLE: EMOTIONAL BREAKTHROUGHS

Consider the case of Emily, who found solace in listening to her heartbeat during therapy. Initially overwhelmed by feelings of fear and isolation, Emily gradually developed emotional resilience. As she engaged with her heartbeat, she stated, "It's like I'm learning to be okay with the unknown." This sentiment encapsulates the transformative power of MHbT, enabling patients to navigate their emotional landscapes more effectively.

Various case studies have also highlighted the significance of family involvement in MHbT. Joint sessions where family members listen to a loved one's heartbeat create opportunities for emotional intimacy and shared healing. By fostering open communication and connection, MHbT strengthens the bonds between family members, enabling them to support one another through difficult times.

We must also remember that the role of community in providing support cannot be overstated. Family members who actively participate in MHbT sessions report feeling a renewed sense of purpose and connection. This communal approach helps alleviate feelings of isolation and allows families to share their experiences, reinforcing the notion that they are not alone in their journey.

As healthcare continues to evolve, the integration of MHbT into holistic care models presents an opportunity to address the emotional and spiritual needs of patients more effectively. By recognizing the importance of the heart as a symbol of life, connection, and continuity, healthcare providers can create environments that foster emotional healing.

To effectively integrate MHbT into patient care plans, practitioners must:

- *Assess Emotional Needs*: Conduct thorough assessments to identify patients' emotional and spiritual needs.
- *Set Clear Objectives*: Define specific goals for MHbT sessions, such as reducing anxiety or fostering family connections.
- *Collaborate with Interdisciplinary Teams*: Work alongside social workers, psychologists, and spiritual care providers to ensure a comprehensive approach to care.

Access to MHbT must be prioritized, particularly for underserved populations. Community-based programs can extend the reach of this therapy, ensuring that individuals and families facing terminal illnesses have access to emotional support and healing.

- *Develop Partnerships*: Collaborate with community organizations to create MHbT workshops and support groups. These partnerships can enhance resource sharing and community engagement.
- *Utilize Technology*: Explore telehealth options to provide remote MHbT sessions for individuals unable to access in-person care. Online platforms can help facilitate connections and offer resources to patients and families.

FINAL REFLECTIONS: THE HEARTBEAT OF HEALING

As we draw this exploration of Meditative Heartbeat Therapy (MHbT) to a close, it is essential to reflect on its transformative potential within hospice and palliative care. The journey through illness, particularly in the context of terminal conditions, is fraught with emotional complexities. MHbT offers a compassionate response to these challenges, providing individuals and families with tools to navigate their feelings, foster connection, and find meaning amidst uncertainty.

At its core, MHbT emphasizes the profound human connection inherent in the experience of listening to one's heartbeat. This connection serves as a reminder that we are not alone in our struggles, even in the face of mortality. The heartbeat transcends words, providing a rhythm that embodies life itself—a constant reminder of our shared humanity.

The integration of MHbT into healthcare practices promotes a culture of compassion and empathy. By prioritizing emotional and spiritual well-being, practitioners can create environments that support healing on multiple levels. As healthcare professionals embrace this holistic approach, they can foster stronger connections with patients and their families, ultimately enhancing the quality of care provided.

As we look to the future, it is vital to remain open to the possibilities that lie ahead for MHbT. With continued research, technological advancements, and community engagement, we can envision a future where MHbT becomes an integral part of patient care across diverse settings.

As practitioners, patients, and families continue to embrace the power of heartbeat awareness, we can create a more compassionate healthcare system—one that honors the emotional and spiritual dimensions of the human experience.

The journey of Meditative Heartbeat Therapy (MHbT) is just beginning. As we stand at the crossroads of innovation and compassion, we have an opportunity to shape the future of healthcare. By integrating MHbT into our practices, we can honor the heart's rhythm as a powerful symbol of life, connection, and healing.

We invite healthcare practitioners, researchers, and community leaders to join us in this mission. Together, we can ensure that the transformative potential of MHbT reaches those who need it most, fostering emotional resilience and spiritual peace for individuals and families facing the profound challenges of terminal illness.

Throughout this text, we have explored the profound potential of Meditative Heartbeat Therapy as a transformative tool in palliative and end-of-life care. These therapies remind us that healing is not confined to curing the body—it is about creating moments of presence, connection, and peace that transcend physical boundaries.

At the heart of this work is the recognition of the patient as a whole person, whose needs extend beyond the physical to encompass emotional, spiritual, and relational dimensions. The steady rhythm of the heartbeat offers a universal anchor, a constant reminder of the resilience of life, even in its final stages. MHbT becomes more than a therapy—it becomes a pathway to dignity and comfort, helping patients navigate their journey with grace.

This book is not only a guide for practitioners but also a call to reimagine what compassionate care can be. It challenges us to integrate science, spirituality, and humanity, creating a holistic framework that places patients and families at the center of care. By weaving together these modalities, we open new possibilities for relief, reflection, and meaning, offering tools that honor the individuality of every patient.

As we move forward, let us carry the principles of presence, connection, and intention into all aspects of care. Whether we are practitioners, caregivers, or patients ourselves, we are all part of the rhythm of healing—a rhythm that echoes through every heartbeat, reminding us of the shared humanity that binds us.

As this journey draws to a close, we offer these ten rhythms to carry forward in your heart. They are not a replacement for the full depth of this work, but rather a gentle refrain—a quiet melody you may hum when the book ends. Each insight here is a heartbeat of wisdom: a simple song of presence, compassion, and care to hold close in the days ahead. Let these truths be like a steady breath or a quiet beat, grounding you and guiding you on the path ahead.

- *Presence is a gift*: listening with your full attention often heals more than words or solutions ever could.
- *The heartbeat is a teacher*: each pulse reminds us that emotions ebb and flow and that simply being here, alive and present, is enough.
- *Find sacred ritual in simplicity*: a shared breath or the touch of a hand on a chest can become a holy moment of comfort and connection.

- *Trust the body's wisdom*: in every beat and breath, our flesh and spirit speak together; honoring them brings insight, agency, and peace.
- *Embrace stillness*: compassion often lives in the quiet pause, where your gentle presence becomes the very medicine.
- *Care for yourself, too*: remember your own heartbeat with the same kindness you offer others, affirming that you are worthy of presence and love.
- *Celebrate connection*: your pulse echoes in the rhythms of all those you love — those who came before you and those who will follow, uniting you in the great human song.
- *Slow down*: in a hurried world, healing unfolds in the gentle rhythm of breath. Cultivate patience and presence as your guides.
- *Seek meaning in the moment*: each heartbeat invites you to explore life's mysteries with courage and curiosity, finding purpose and peace even in uncertainty.
- *Hold each heartbeat as sacred*: the simple act of listening is itself an act of love and reverence, honoring life and the grace of care in every moment.

May each breath and heartbeat bless your continued journey of presence and care.

BIBLIOGRAPHY

- Chadwick, Paul, et al. "Mindfulness Groups in Palliative Care: A Pilot Qualitative Study." *Palliative Medicine*, vol. 22, no. 7, 2008, pp. 780–786.
- Cohen, Sheldon, Denise Janicki-Deverts, and Gregory E. Miller. "Psychological Stress and Disease." *JAMA*, vol. 298, no. 14, 2007, pp. 1685–1687.
- Creswell, J. David, and Emily K. Lindsay. "How Mindfulness Improves Emotion Regulation: A Neurobiological Perspective." *Current Directions in Psychological Science*, vol. 23, no. 1, 2014, pp. 14–20.
- Elder, Susan, and James Elder. *The Healing Heart: A Guide to Using Your Heartbeat to Heal*. [Publisher Unknown], 2017.
- Fisher, Julie. *Mindful Compassion: Using the Power of Mindfulness and Compassion to Transform Your Life*. Shambhala, 2013.
- Germer, Christopher K., and Ronald D. Siegel. *Wisdom and Compassion in Psychotherapy: Cultivating Well-Being in Your Clients and Yourself*. Guilford Press, 2012.
- Hölzel, Britta K., et al. "Mindfulness Practice Leads to Increases in Regional Brain Gray Matter Density." *Psychiatry Research: Neuroimaging*, vol. 191, no. 1, 2011, pp. 36–43.
- Jaffray, Linda, et al. "Evaluating the Effects of Mindfulness-Based Interventions for Informal Palliative Caregivers: A Systematic Literature Review." *Palliative Medicine*, vol. 30, no. 2, 2016, pp. 117–131.
- Kabat-Zinn, Jon. *Full Catastrophe Living: Using the Wisdom of Your Body and Mind to Face Stress, Pain, and Illness*. Delacorte Press, 1990.
- Latorraca, Carolina de Oliveira Cruz, et al. "Mindfulness for Palliative Care Patients: A Systematic Review of Randomized Controlled Trials." *International Journal of Clinical Practice*, vol. 72, 2017, e13034.

Appendix

PRACTICAL TOOLS AND WORKBOOKS
FOR MEDITATIVE HEARTBEAT THERAPY

In the practice of Meditative Heartbeat Therapy (MHbT), having practical tools and resources is essential for both practitioners and patients. These resources help structure the therapy sessions, facilitate emotional exploration, and encourage reflection. This chapter provides a comprehensive overview of workbooks, exercises, and templates designed to enhance the MHbT experience, making it accessible and effective for diverse populations.

TOOLS FOR PRACTITIONERS:
IMPLEMENTING MHBT EFFECTIVELY

Developing a clear structure for each MHbT session is vital for both the practitioner and the patient. Below are templates that practitioners can use to guide sessions effectively.

Template 1: Individual MHbT Session Outline

1. *Opening (5 minutes)*
   - Greet the patient and establish a comfortable environment.

- Briefly discuss the patient's emotional state and any concerns they wish to address.

2. *Grounding Exercise (10 minutes)*
   - Begin with breath awareness to help the patient relax.
   - Use guided imagery to help them visualize a safe and calming space.

3. *Heartbeat Listening (15 minutes)*
   - Record the patient's heartbeat and play it back.
   - Encourage the patient to focus solely on the sound, observing any emotions or thoughts that arise.

4. *Reflective Discussion (15 minutes)*
   - Ask the patient open-ended questions about their experience:
     - "What emotions did you notice while listening to your heartbeat?"
     - "How does your heartbeat relate to your current feelings?"

5. *Closing Reflection (5 minutes)*
   - Summarize the session and highlight key insights.
   - Provide the patient with any relevant journaling prompts for self-reflection after the session.

Template 2: Family MHbT Session Outline

1. *Introduction (5 minutes)*
   - Welcome family members and establish a supportive environment.
   - Discuss the goals of the session.

2. *Joint Grounding Exercise (10 minutes)*
   - Engage the family in synchronized breathing exercises.
   - Encourage them to connect with each other and feel the shared space.

3. *Heartbeat Listening (15 minutes)*
   - Use the recording of the patient's heartbeat for family members to listen to together.

- ○ Create a moment of silence to foster emotional connection.

4. *Family Reflection (15 minutes)*
    - ○ Invite family members to share their feelings about the experience.
    - ○ Use reflective questions to guide the discussion:
        - ▪ "What did listening to the heartbeat evoke for each of you?"
        - ▪ "How can this experience help you support one another?"

5. *Closing Ceremony (5 minutes)*
    - ○ Offer a closing ritual, such as a moment of silence or sharing a group affirmation.
    - ○ Encourage ongoing communication and support within the family.

JOURNALING AND REFLECTION PROMPTS

Journaling serves as a powerful tool for patients and families to process their emotions and reflect on their experiences. Below are specific prompts designed to accompany MHbT sessions:

1. *Reflecting on Heartbeat Awareness*
    - ○ "What emotions surfaced while listening to my heartbeat? How did it make me feel?"
    - ○ "Did I notice any physical sensations in my body while I listened? What were they?"

2. *Exploring Memories and Legacy*
    - ○ "What life lessons do I want to share with my loved ones?"
    - ○ "How do I want to be remembered, and what do I wish to leave behind?"

3. *Coping with Emotions*
    - ○ "When I feel anxious, how does my heartbeat change? What strategies can I use to calm myself?"

○ "What affirmations or positive thoughts can I focus on during moments of distress?"

JOURNALING PROMPTS FOR FAMILIES

1. *Shared Reflections*
   ○ "What did I learn about my loved one during this session?"
   ○ "How can we better support each other through this journey?"
2. *Expressing Gratitude*
   ○ "What moments of joy or connection have I shared with my loved one that I cherish?"
   ○ "How can I express my love and appreciation to them daily?"
3. *Facing Challenges Together*
   ○ "What fears do I have about the end of life, and how can we confront these fears as a family?"
   ○ "How can we create a supportive environment for open communication?"

www.ingramcontent.com/pod-product-compliance
Lightning Source LLC
Chambersburg PA
CBHW020531270326
41927CB00006B/528